W9-CHS-707

# Medicare in the
# Twenty-first Century

# Medicare in the Twenty-first Century

## Seeking Fair and Efficient Reform

Robert B. Helms, editor

The AEI Press

Publisher for the American Enterprise Institute
WASHINGTON, D.C.

*1999*

Available in the United States from the AEI Press, c/o Publisher Resources Inc., 1224 Heil Quaker Blvd., P. O. Box 7001, La Vergne, TN 37086-7001. To order, call 1-800-269-6267. Distributed outside the United States by arrangement with Eurospan, 3 Henrietta Street, London WC2E 8LU, England.

**Library of Congress Cataloging-in-Publication Data**
Medicare in the twenty-first century : seeking fair and efficient
  reform / Robert B. Helms, editor.
    p.  cm.
  Includes bibliographical references and index.
  ISBN 0-8447-4117-5 (cloth : alk. paper). — ISBN 0-8447-4118-3
  (paper : alk. paper)
  1. Medicare.
  RA412.3.M436      1999
  368.4'00973—dc21                                              99-40486
                                                                    CIP


1 3 5 7 9 10 8 6 4 2

© 1999 by the American Enterprise Institute for Public Policy Research, Washington, D.C. All rights reserved. No part of this publication may be used or reproduced in any manner whatsoever without permission in writing from the American Enterprise Institute except in the case of brief quotations embodied in news articles, critical articles, or reviews. The views expressed in the publications of the American Enterprise Institute are those of the authors and do not necessarily reflect the views of the staff, advisory panels, officers, or trustees of AEI.

The AEI Press
Publisher for the American Enterprise Institute
1150 17th Street, N.W., Washington, D.C. 20036

*Printed in the United States of America*

# Contents

# Contributors

JOSEPH R. ANTOS is the assistant director for health and human resources—the division providing Congress with analyses of proposed changes to federal programs and policies in areas such as health, income security, education, employment, and housing—at the Congressional Budget Office. He was the director of the Office of Research and Demonstrations and the deputy director of the Office of the Actuary at the Health Care Financing Administration. Mr. Antos was the deputy chief of staff and the principal deputy assistant secretary for management and budget at the Department of Health and Human Services.

LINDA BILHEIMER is the deputy assistant director for health at the Congressional Budget Office. She directs a team of economists who analyze the budgetary and policy consequences of legislative proposals for health care with a focus on their cost implications for the federal government and the private sector. Before joining the CBO in 1991, Ms. Bilheimer was a senior researcher at Mathematica Policy Research, and, from 1982 to 1987, she was the director of health statistics and epidemiology in the Arkansas Department of Health.

BRYAN DOWD is an associate professor in the Institute for Health Services Research in the School of Public Health at the University of Minnesota and the director of graduate studies for the master of science program in health services research and policy. Mr. Dowd's primary research interests are markets for health insurance and health care services and the evaluation of nonexperimental data. His recent research includes studies of health plan choice, resource use, and health status of Medicare beneficiaries in the Twin Cities; a comparison of TEFRA-risks and social HMO enrollees; and a national survey of large public employers to examine their health insurance purchasing practices. With Roger Feldman and Jon Christianson, he wrote *Competitive Pricing for Medicare* (AEI Press, 1996).

ROGER FELDMAN is the Blue Cross Professor of Health Insurance at the University of Minnesota. He directed one of the four national research centers sponsored by the Health Care Financing Administration and was a senior staff member of the Council of Economic Advisers, where he was lead author of one chapter of the *1985 Economic Report of the President*. Mr. Feldman is on the editorial board of *Inquiry* and is a regular contributor to health services research and economics journals. His research interests include competition among health care providers and health maintenance organizations. With Bryan Dowd and Jon Christianson, Mr. Feldman wrote *Competitive Pricing for Medicare* (AEI Press, 1996). He is working on a study of horizontal mergers among hospitals.

WALTON FRANCIS is a self-employed economist and analyst. He was an economist and policy analyst in the Office of the Assistant Secretary for Planning and Evaluation at the Department of Health and Human Services. As the director of the Division of Policy and Regulatory Analysis, he reviewed regulatory proposals to analyze their economic effects and minimize unnecessary burdens, and he designed and evaluated policy proposals on health, income supports, social services, and management problems. He has written on managed health care and retirement benefits and is a leading expert on the Federal Employees Health Benefits Program. Mr. Francis pioneered the systematic comparison of health insurance plans from a consumer perspective and continues as the author of the annual *Checkbook's Guide to Health Insurance Plans for Federal Employees*.

H. E. FRECH III is a professor of economics at the University of California at Santa Barbara, an adjunct scholar at AEI, and an adjunct professor at Sciences Po de Paris. He has been a visiting professor at the University of Chicago and at Harvard University. From 1970 to 1972 Mr. Frech was an economist with the Department of Health, Education, and Welfare. He has published more than ninety articles and books on industrial organization, health economics, and other topics. Mr. Frech is the author of *Competition and Monopoly in Medical Care* (AEI Press, 1996) and, with Richard D. Miller, Jr., *The Productivity of Health Care and Pharmaceuticals: An International Comparison* (AEI Press, 1999).

ROBERT B. HELMS is a resident scholar and the director of health policy studies at the American Enterprise Institute. He has written and lectured extensively on health policy, health economics, and pharmaceutical economic issues. Mr. Helms participates in the Consensus Group, an informal task force that is developing market-oriented health reform concepts, and is on the National Academy of Social Insurance's study panel on long-term Medicare financing. From 1981 to 1989, he was the assistant secretary for planning and evaluation and deputy assistant secretary for health policy in the Department of Health and Human Services. Mr. Helms is the editor of several AEI publications on health policy in addition to this volume: *American Health Policy: Critical Issues for Reform; Health Policy Reform: Competition and Controls; Health Care Policy and Politics: Lessons from Four Countries;* and *Competitive Strategies in the Pharmaceutical Industry.*

LEN M. NICHOLS joined the health policy center at the Urban Institute in November 1994. His research focuses on various aspects of markets and health reform: insurance market regulation; the elasticity of demand for health insurance; alternative risk-pooling arrangements; tax incentives and health insurance purchase decisions; health insurance purchasing cooperatives; and private insurance options for Medicare. Mr. Nichols was the senior adviser for health policy at the Office of Management and Budget in 1993–1994, when he managed and coordinated cost and revenue estimations for President Clinton's Health Security Act and its congressional successors. He was a visiting public health service fellow at the Agency for Health Care Policy and Research in 1991–1992, and an associate professor and chairman of the Economics Department at Wellesley College, where he taught from 1980 to 1991. Mr. Nichols is a member of the Competitive Pricing Advisory Commission (CPAC) for the Medicare program.

MARK V. PAULY is a professor of health care systems, insurance and risk management, and public policy and management at the Wharton School, professor of economics at the School of Arts and Sciences, and Bendheim

Professor at the University of Pennsylvania. He is also a member of the Institute of Medicine and an adjunct scholar of the American Enterprise Institute. Mr. Pauly was the director of research and the executive director at the Leonard Davis Institute of Health Economics, a visiting research fellow at the International Institute of Management, a commissioner on the Physician Payment Review Commission, and a professor of economics at Northwestern University. He is the author of *Pooling Health Insurance Risks*, with Bradley Herring (AEI Press, 1999), *Financing Long-Term Care: What Should Be the Government's Role?* with Peter Zweifel (AEI Press, 1996), *An Analysis of Medical Savings Accounts: Do Two Wrongs Make a Right?* (AEI Press, 1994), and *Responsible National Health Insurance*, with Patricia Danzon, Paul Feldstein, and John Hoff (AEI Press, 1992).

ANDREW J. RETTENMAIER is a research associate at the Private Enterprise Research Center of Texas A&M University. His primary research areas are labor economics and public policy economics. Mr. Rettenmaier and PERC's director, Thomas R. Saving, have presented their Medicare reform proposal to U.S. Senate subcommittees and to the National Bipartisan Commission on the Future of Medicare. Their proposal has also been featured in the *Wall Street Journal, New England Journal of Medicine, Houston Chronicle,* and *Dallas Morning News*. Mr. Rettenmaier is the coauthor of *The Economics of Medicare Reform* (Upjohn Institute for Employment Research, forthcoming) and an editor of *Medicare Reform: Issues and Answers* (University of Chicago Press, forthcoming).

THOMAS R. SAVING is the director of the Private Enterprise Research Center, a University Distinguished Professor of Economics, and the Jeff Montgomery Professor of Economics at Texas A&M University. His current research emphasis is on the benefit of markets in solving the pressing issues in health care. Mr. Saving was the president of the Western Economics Association and the Southern Economics Association, and he was on the faculties of the University of Washington and Michigan State University. He is the author of two books on monetary theory and of more than forty articles on antitrust and monetary economics, health economics, the theory of the banking firm, and the general theory of the firm and markets.

# *1*

# *Introduction*

## Robert B. Helms

M any Americans are trying to ignore the issue of saving the popular Medicare program. Although the National Bipartisan Commission on the Future of Medicare (established by Congress as part of the Balanced Budget Act of 1997) recently spent a year trying to devise a reform plan, Medicare reform is receiving relatively little attention from politicians and the press. In a recent poll, only 39 percent of Americans knew that the Medicare commission existed (Kaiser Family Foundation 1998). Since the 1996 national elections, when both major political parties featured Medicare in a series of unnerving political advertisements, political strategists have been advising their candidate-clients not to take the political risk of talking about Medicare. Public opinion polls indicate that while Medicare is a popular program, its reform is not a leading concern for most people (KFF-Harvard 1999).

This inattention to the problems besetting Medicare cannot continue. Medicare is the second largest government entitlement program; it provides medical care to 39 million elderly and disabled people, with annual expenditures of approximately $214 billion in 1998, or 2.65 percent of the gross domestic product. According to the expert opinions of actuaries, academics, and health policy researchers, Medicare cannot survive the first half of the twenty-first century without major reforms. In their most recent report, the trustees of the Medicare trust funds project that the hospital insurance (HI) trust fund, which covers hospital care, will run out of funds in 2015, and the supplementary medical insurance (SMI) trust fund, which pays for physician and other outpatient services, will require increasing subsidies from general revenues to cover its expenses (Board of Trustees, HI 1999, 2; Board of Trustees, SMI 1999, 2). Program expenditures for the HI and SMI programs combined are projected to increase to 3.04 percent of GDP in 2010 and to 4.88 percent in 2030 (Board of Trustees, HI 1999, 76). Meanwhile, neither the number of workers nor the taxes that they pay will grow nearly as fast as the number of Medicare enrollees and the cost of their medical care (Board of Trustees, HI 1999, 2–3).

Approximately 9.6 million people work in the health sector. Given the importance of medical care for the aged and disabled, most of these professionals are directly affected by the Medicare program (Census Bureau 1997, 122). From almost any perspective, Medicare cannot be ignored—yet, it is.

The authors of this volume take as a given the necessity of Medicare reform, a reform that will require intense political debate before a compromise of some sort is reached. The timing of this debate is uncertain but will likely be driven by the cycle of presidential and congressional elections, the declining balances of the Part A trust fund, and the continuing aging of the baby boom generation, which becomes eligible for Medicare after 2010.

Another factor in Medicare reform will be the debate about Social Security reform. Since Medicare was passed as an amendment to the Social Security Act (Helms 1999), it shares many common features with Social Security in its operation, financing, and plans for reform. Although the Medicare benefit is more complicated than the Social Security cash benefit, both programs are substantially funded by a commonly administered payroll tax, and both programs provide benefits to the same cohorts of people. Because both programs face significant long-term deficits, as well as consume a growing portion of the federal budget, any discussion of reform of one program must invariably involve the other (Weaver forthcoming; Peterson 1996; Robertson 1997). In 1997, federal spending on Social Security and Medicare (Parts A and B) amounted to $570 billion, or one-third of the entire federal budget. The Congressional Budget Office estimates that, by 2030, spending on these two programs will account for half of all federal spending (CBO 1998a, 70, and b, xvi).

This volume does not seek consensus about how to reform Medicare. But the authors do share one attribute: they have completed serious research and have done serious thinking about how to improve Medicare. The authors were asked for relatively short essays about program reform. They were instructed to spend little time on the wrongs with the current program and to demonstrate instead how Medicare could be made more efficient and maintain fairness to all those affected. As the resulting chapters show, the disagreement regarding the principles of reform continues even among those who think about incentives and share the common objective of improving Medicare's efficiency.

## Fairness and Efficiency

Fairness and efficiency are at the heart of the political debate about Medicare reform. The discussion is complicated by the fact that fairness and efficiency mean different things to different people. Many competing interests are involved: the young and the old, taxpayers and beneficiaries, patients and providers, those who stand to gain or lose depending on the nature of the reforms. What may seem fair to one group of people may seem unfair to another. Ultimately this concern for fairness and the economic reality of Medicare's financing problems are the two forces that will drive this debate.

**The Political Imperative.** For a better understanding of the concern for fairness that continually exerts its influence in all political debates, let us consider first one future scenario that is unlikely to meet anyone's definition of either fairness or efficiency: a continuation of the status quo. In essence this is what the Medicare actuaries estimate each year and include in the annual trustees' report. These projections are their best guess about what will happen to the program under varying economic and demographic assumptions if no changes are made in the laws governing Medicare. While the 1999 report indicates some improvement over 1998, the following quotations illustrate the basic imbalance of current-law Medicare:

On the Part A side, the actuaries say:

There are expected to be 3.6 workers per HI beneficiary when the baby boom generation begins to reach age 65 in 2010. Then the worker/beneficiary ratio is expected to rapidly decline to 2.3 in 2030 as the last of the baby boomers reaches age 65. . . . HI expenditures are projected to grow rapidly as a fraction of workers' earnings, from 3.2 percent in 1998 to 6.8 percent in 2070. As a fraction of the Gross Domestic Product (GDP), expenditures would grow somewhat more slowly, from 1.6 percent in 1998 to 3.0 percent in 2070. . . . Projected HI tax income would meet only a declining share of expenditures under present law. Tax income is expected to equal 97 percent of expenditures in 1999 and 86 percent in 2015 (when the fund is estimated to be depleted), and would cover about one-half of costs 75 years from now. (Board of Trustees, HI 1999, 2)

For Part B, the actuaries say:

SMI benefits have been growing rapidly although rates of growth have moderated in recent years. Even so, outlays have increased 41 percent over the last 5 years (33 percent on a per-beneficiary basis). During this period the program grew about 9 percent faster than the economy as a whole, despite efforts to control SMI costs. . . . SMI expenditures are expected to continue to grow faster than the economy as a whole. SMI outlays were less than 1 percent of the Gross Domestic Product (GDP) in 1998 and are projected to grow to about 2.7 percent by 2070. (Board of Trustees, SMI, 1999, 2)

Since these are actuarial estimates about future events, there is no guarantee of complete accuracy. But few experts doubt that the figures will be far from the mark. Unforeseen events that are worse than expected (for example, an economic recession, an unexpected disease outbreak, a new expensive medical technology) are more likely than unforeseen events for the better (for example, unexpected economic growth, an unexpected improvement in the health of the elderly, large savings in costs from the increased use of the new Medicare+Choice options added in the Balanced Budget Act, or a new medical technology that reduces the cost of treatment). The shortfalls in projected revenues compared with the projected expenditures in the second and third decades of the next century are so large that minor adjustments to the actuaries' basic assumptions probably cannot substantially change the picture. Further, many experts believe that the intermediate projections are too optimistic and that the pessimistic projections are more likely to occur (King 1996).

In the unlikely event that no congressional action changes either the revenue or expenditures, the Health Care Financing Administration would have no authority to continue paying Medicare claims once the HI trust fund became exhausted. Based on the rate of inflow of payroll taxes, HCFA might decide to pay some fraction of each claim, but this action would not be likely to save the program for long because of two probable reactions from hospitals and physicians submitting claims: (1) an increase in the volume of claims submitted as providers seek to make up for the missing revenue and (2) a refusal by many providers to continue treating at least some Medicare patients if the government refused to pay the full legal amount for each claim. Such a situation would not be politically acceptable and would certainly not meet anyone's definition of fairness or efficiency. These circumstances would deny both needed medical services to Medicare recipients and payments to medical professionals and institutions providing that care.

A probable variation on this scenario, based on past congressional actions, finds Congress moving to reduce Medicare payments for services without doing anything to reform the program's fundamental structure (CBO 1997; Kahn and Kuttner 1999). Tighter price controls might extend the life of the HI trust fund for a few years but would be politically unacceptable, as the baby boom generation begins to join Medicare after 2010 and as the level of access and quality begins to deteriorate because of reduced payments.[1] Results would include increasingly wasteful economic behavior by providers and patients, less medical care for eligible Medicare recipients, and payments to providers that they would consider unfair.

But fairness means not merely keeping the Medicare program operating. While Medicare beneficiaries are required to pay some out-of-pocket expenses, including Part B premiums and copayments, taxpayers support a significant portion of the health expenses of the elderly and disabled (HCFA 1998). In 1998, taxpayers paid $124 billion in payroll taxes to finance Part A and an additional $60 billion in income taxes to fund Part B through general revenues, that is, 88 percent of the Part A income and 73 percent of the Part B income (Board of Trustees, HI 1999, 34; Board of Trustees, SMI 1999, 28). Relatively few working elderly still pay Medicare and income taxes; younger taxpayers provide the majority of the funding for Medicare. And as the baby boom generation ages and the proportion of the population older than sixty-five mushrooms, this disproportionate burden on the young will only increase. In 1998, there were nearly 3.9 workers per Medicare beneficiary. In 2010, when the first baby boomers join the Medicare rolls, this proportion will drop to 3.6 and will decline rapidly thereafter, as it falls to only 2.3 in 2030, when the last baby boomers reach age sixty-five (Board of Trustees, HI 1999, 2, 13).

This aspect of fairness is usually referred to as intergenerational equity, a term associated with the empirical work of Larry Kotlikoff (Gokhale and Kotlikoff 1998; Kotlikoff 1992; Auerbach, Gokhale, and Kotlikoff 1991). Discussion of this aspect of fairness is dominated by the liabilities placed on future generations of workers by the current method of financing. Gokhale and Kotlikoff (1998) find that those now middle-aged and older will fare quite well under the present system regarding the present value of their taxes in comparison with the present value of expected Medicare benefits, while newborns and future generations of workers face substantial losses. To achieve balance between the present value of benefits and that of taxes, Gokhale and Kotlikoff estimate that the Medicare program would have to be cut today by a permanent 68 percent. In another five years, the program would have to be cut by a permanent 78 percent, and by 2016 even the total elimination of the program could not achieve generational balance (Gokhale and Kotlikoff 1998, 18).

The Congressional Budget Office has made similar calculations in estimating the net transfers under Medicare for single men and women with average earnings by discounting the value of future lifetime benefits and lifetime taxes.[2] The net transfer for a single man with average earnings on reaching age sixty-five in 1985 is $32,222—this is the difference between the present value of the benefits that he could expect to receive from Medicare and the total lifetime taxes that he paid into the system. Stated another way, the present value of his total lifetime taxes is only 29 percent of his lifetime benefits. For men reaching age sixty-five in 1995 and 2005, the net transfers are even larger: $51,813 and $71,868, respectively. For women, who have longer life expectancies, the transfers are greater than for men. The net transfers were $41,355 for the 1985 retiree, $68,777 for the 1995 retiree, and $91,594 for a single women with average earnings retiring in 2005. These calculations are for individuals who qualify for Medicare benefits on the basis of their own work. But up to 20 percent of Medicare beneficiaries qualify on the basis of their spouse's work history; for these people, net lifetime transfers would be substantially higher because they have paid little or no HI taxes (Committee on Ways and Means 1998, 126).

Looked at in this way, the present method of financing Medicare obviously cannot be sustained in the next century. While income and payroll taxes affect incentives differently, substantial increases in either would significantly diminish the incentives of taxpayers. For example, high marginal rates of income taxation encourage tax cheating and erode much of the incentive to earn additional income. High rates of payroll taxes fall disproportionately on younger workers, shrink employment, and diminish incentives to work.

Another aspect of fairness with a strong role in the Medicare debate is the financial burden imposed on the elderly by their relatively high use of medical services. The use and the expense of medical care are strongly related to age. In 1996, average yearly Medicare expenditures for those aged eighty-five and older were estimated at $7,132, nearly twice the average yearly expenditures for beneficiaries aged sixty-five to sixty-nine (Moon 1997). Out-of-pocket expenditures for drugs and chronic health conditions not covered by Medicare also increase with age. When compared with the typically declining income of the elderly, the financial burden of medical expenses seems to increase with age. However, when compared with the increasing wealth of the elderly, the burden looks more manageable (Weicher 1995, 1997; National Bipartisan Commission 1998).

These two considerations of the burden of medical expenditures, first on taxpayers and then on the elderly, illustrate the importance of fairness in the Medicare reform debate. Policies that seem fair to the young will not be considered by many as fair to the elderly because more moderate taxes on active workers mean reduced benefits and increased financial obligations for Medicare recipients. Political theory might suggest that political compromise will induce politicians to settle on a solution that minimizes the damage to all affected groups—a solution that no one seems to be happy about but that wins out because conditions demand a solution and the compromise seems better than prolonging the debate.

**The Economic Imperative.** Economists are fond of saying that there is no free lunch. When talking about Medicare, perhaps we should add "especially for politicians." The political struggle to balance the interests of large groups of voters must take into account the economic reality of Medicare financing. Political debates that become a competition between candidates to see who can offer the most in additional benefits tend to obscure the real economic costs of the Medicare program. In the most fundamental sense, any service provided to a Medicare recipient uses up real economic resources that cannot be used for other purposes. Even in a segment of the economy with relatively large volunteer and philanthropic inputs, most nurses, physicians, and other medical personnel must be paid for the value of their time and training. Investments in research and development and in capital structures require rates of return sufficient to divert these resources to medical uses. And, in terms of the federal budget, tax resources devoted to entitlement programs such as Medicare reduce the resources that are available for other discretionary parts of the budget (CBO 1998a). Everything has a cost, but political debates often proceed with slight acknowledgment of elementary economic reality.

How bad is the economic plight facing Medicare? There is little disagreement with the official government projections that the current program with its current tax base and current benefits cannot survive through the second decade of the next century. The main disagreement about the actuarial projections is that the basic economic assumptions are too optimistic (Reischauer 1997; Wilensky and Newhouse 1999). Additionally, there is substantial disagreement about how to reform the system, especially how to restructure consumer and provider incentives and the capacity of various groups of taxpayers to give up the real resources necessary to keep the program going (Moon 1999). This volume reflects some of that disagreement.

Not only is there an economic imperative to reform Medicare: there is an economic imperative to improve the efficiency of the program. Based on their research about the efficiency of medical markets, the authors of this volume are seeking in these essays to improve both the efficiency and the fairness of the program. What do we mean by economic efficiency? It is not simply the reduction of costs, since, as costs are reduced, the owners of labor and capital have incentives at some point to divert their resources away from medical care, so that the benefits actually received by consumers are also reduced. Neither is economic efficiency the maximization of medical benefits to patients. As more resources are added to improve medical benefits, at some point the value of the additional benefits becomes less than the value placed on nonmedical benefits that must be given up. Nor is economic efficiency the payment of the maximum amount to those who supply the inputs to medical care, the physicians, nurses, and managers who work in the system and those investors who supply the capital for physical facilities and medical equipment and products. As more is paid for inputs, at some point the additional output produced becomes less than the value of the alternative products and services that could otherwise have been produced.

The common factor of all these misleading evaluations is the notion of maximizing some objective without any constraints. In the real world, a balance must be reached among competing objectives. The concept of economic efficiency is defined in terms of a balance at the margin: it is achieved when the marginal cost of producing an additional unit of output is just equal to the marginal benefit of that output as evaluated by consumers. The formal theory of economic efficiency, commonly referred to as welfare economics, also shows how nonmarket distortions such as price controls, tax subsidies, cost-increasing regulation, or producers' collusive behavior can prevent economic efficiency and impose dead-weight losses on the economy.

Tom Rice (1998) has recently, and vigorously, attacked the application of this formal theory to medical markets and health policy; Martin Gaynor and William Vogt (1997), Mark Pauly (1997, 467–73), and Bryan Dowd (1999, 266–69) have ably defended that use. This volume does not attempt to settle the largely theoretical dispute but does proceed with the notion that the concept of economic efficiency can contribute to the search for efficient Medicare reform.

What is most misunderstood about the concept of economic efficiency is its emphasis on efficient adjustment to changing consumer preferences and production technology. The beauty of the concept is in the seeking. Economic efficiency does not imply that each consumer gets everything he wants, but it does imply that an economic system with the correct incentives will continually adjust itself to account for changing consumer demands and changing conditions in the production of the desired output. If a new medical technology allows for cheaper production of an existing medical service or of a new medical procedure desired by consumers, those seeking their own gain (Smith 1937) will ensure that the new technology is developed, tested, and introduced into the market at the most efficient rate.[3] Even if we cannot empirically identify an efficient medical market, the theory tells us that policies that allow market forces to adjust market prices continually will induce all market participants to seek to improve the cost-effectiveness of their decisions, consumers to seek value in the purchase of medical goods and services, and producers to seek to produce what consumers want with the most efficient technologies and combinations of inputs. An improvement in economic efficiency means that we get more of what we want for the resources that we give up, a worthy goal in Medicare reform.

Still, as these essays show, there is much room for improvement. Neither the present Medicare program nor the U.S. health care system within which it operates is a model of efficiency. Major impediments to efficiency include the following:

- cost-sharing features whose effectiveness has been seriously eroded by medical inflation during Medicare's thirty-four-year history
- administered hospital and physician price controls that inhibit the ability of the market to ration care and to create incentives for improved quality
- a system of mandated benefits that reduces the incentives of providers and patients to consider the cost-effectiveness of both old and new technologies and procedures
- an antiquated system of paying for managed care that inhibits the growth and increases the costs of this method of organizing and delivering care and causes severe geographical distortions in payment rates and enrollment
- an open-ended funding mechanism for Part B that places unlimited liabilities on the general U.S. budget and reduces the incentives of all participants (patients, providers, program administrators, and politicians) to control the cost of physician care
- payroll financing for Part A that places an increasing burden on younger workers and thereby causes increased unemployment, inefficient employment arrangements, and more workers without health insurance

For various historical and political reasons, Medicare policies cause a number of costly inefficiencies and, as Ted Frech points out in chapter 6, have prevented the program from adopting many of the market innovations found in the private sector.

## A Review of Reform Proposals

The seven essays in this volume trace a logical progression in the history and analysis of the relevant issues. The following summaries are not exhaustive but are intended only to give the reader an indication of the approach and topics of each essay.

**The Bumpy Road.** Chapter 2 provides a comprehensive discussion of reform options. Joseph R. Antos and Linda Bilheimer use recent CBO studies and projections to analyze the inventory of policy reforms that might be considered to correct the financial and structural deficiencies of the current program. They consider the many varieties of reform proposals in three broad categories: (1) policies that reduce costs without improving efficiency, (2) policies that reduce costs and improve program efficiency, and (3) policies that restructure Medicare's financing. A central theme throughout their analysis is the need to address what to do with archaic and dysfunctional aspects of Medicare's basic design. The authors analyze several reforms designed to affect consumer behavior (for example, cost-sharing, vouchers, and more use of managed care). Reductions in provider payments and infusions of new revenue may temporarily improve the status of trust funds, but they would do nothing to change the behavior of beneficiaries, who have little incentive to control their use of services.

The authors' analysis of the Balanced Budget Act of 1997 shows that none of these issues were addressed in a way likely to bring about the fundamental reform necessary for Medicare to survive. They conclude that nothing now guarantees that the expectations of the baby boom generation for the future of Medicare will be met. With 84 percent of Medicare beneficiaries still in the traditional fee-for-service sector, Medicare, in their view, cannot be preserved without fundamental reform.

**Financing.** When compared with the existing and growing body of literature about Medicare, chapter 3 is unique in two ways. First, it starts with a history of issues raised by some key players in the debate leading up to the passage of Medicare in 1965, issues relating to the viability of a system of financing based on payroll taxes. Second, Andrew J. Rettenmaier and Thomas R. Saving concentrate on the financing of Medicare, which, they argue, is generally ignored in the reform debate.

They explain the economic effects of the present system of financing Medicare through a transfer of funds from active workers to retirees and compare this with what would happen if Medicare were prefunded; this is, if current workers were required or induced to save for their medical care after retirement. The authors show that a prefunded system would result in a larger capital stock in the economy than under our present transfer system and that the increased income from this larger capital stock could be used to ease the transition from one system to the other. Rettenmaier and Saving present revenue and cost estimates of a transition to a prefunded system. One alarming implication of their illustration is the importance of starting any transition sooner rather than later.

**Beneficiary Contributions.** In chapter 4 Mark V. Pauly analyzes an issue at the center of the debate about fairness: the ability of higher-income beneficiaries to pay a higher portion of the cost of Medicare. To set the stage, he considers two alternative approaches to reform: the prefunding proposal by Rettenmaier and Saving in chapter 3 and a policy relying on reductions in provider payments. While Pauly sees some advantages to prefunding, he questions both the political viability and the fairness of requiring the middle generation of workers to take on the double burden of paying for the current elderly and to build a fund for their own retirement benefits. He argues that his proposal is compatible with Rettenmaier and Saving's proposal since his would reduce the burden that current policy places on the current generation and the burden expected on the younger generation in future years.

Pauly also argues that there may be some advantages to Medicare from further reductions in provider payments. Given Medicare's large market share, it can act like any large purchaser with market power and can cut provider rates even further, since there is little evidence that providers are refusing to service Medicare beneficiaries at present payment levels. But his principal criticism of both approaches is a lack of improvement in the efficiency of Medicare financing or delivery.

To achieve this improvement, Pauly proposes a system of income- and risk-related vouchers or subsidies to provide more complete coverage for the poorer and sicker while scaling down the coverage for those who are relatively more healthy and wealthy. If the original purpose of Medicare was to help the elderly receive more medical care than they would have been able to afford, the current system is both inefficient and inequitable: it encourages excessive use and redistributes income from the poor to the rich. The author presents data showing that the income of the elderly has grown substantially since 1965; a larger proportion of those on Medicare can pay more of the costs. Medicare is inferior to a progressive income tax as a way to redistribute income, since a uniform medical benefit set to cover the needs of the low-income group will induce the higher-income group to consume excessive care. If Medicare benefits were set to decline with income, gains in efficiency would result from both a reduction in excess consumption and a reduction in the negative effects of the payroll tax on work effort and savings. Pauly points out that a defined contribution that declines with income would be easier to administer than trying to means-test deductibles and cost sharing in the present benefit package.

Chapter 4 also discusses problems presented by the supplementation of Medicare coverage through the purchase of Medigap policies. The extent of such purchasing by higher-income beneficiaries is strong evidence that the present subsidy to these beneficiaries is too large. Pauly argues that Medicare's financial problems are so large that relatively small steps cannot solve the problem; he presents some estimates of the extent of the financial changes required to restore both the efficiency and the soundness of the program. As a strong rationale for his proposal, he states, "Low-income elders need comprehensive insurance coverage more generous than current Medicare, high-income elders need catastrophic coverage at a reasonable price, and middle-class people of all ages need moderate taxes."

**Managing the Market.** Len M. Nichols begins by pointing out that Medicare has become the most popular public program but needs structural repair to fulfill its promises in the twenty-first century. He uses a few equations and some relatively simple data on rates of growth of key variables to illustrate powerfully why controlling the growth of cost per beneficiary is the most promising policy variable for maintaining the quality of services and for keeping tax increases reasonable.

Before giving his prescription for effective competition, Nichols reminds us of some realities of Medicare that will complicate rapid reform. His caveats include these:

- Approximately 16 percent of Medicare enrollees are also enrolled in Medicaid.
- Almost two-thirds of Medicare beneficiaries live in households with incomes below $20,000.
- Of all Medicare beneficiaries, 84 percent participate in the fee-for-service (FFS) part of the program.
- Few managed-care plans participating in Medicare are prepared to care for the chronically ill and disabled elderly.
- Although relatively little is known about how to design effective risk adjusters and competitive bidding practices, both will be necessary for effective competition in Medicare markets.

Nichols assumes that FFS will remain an option for beneficiaries and that competitive bidding will replace the current adjusted average per capita cost (AAPCC) system for paying competing health plans. With the preceding caveats in mind, the author outlines six steps to achieve the value-based purchasing of health insurance:

1. Define benefit packages. Nichols rejects the notion of a single benefit package for everyone but argues that specifying a set of basic benefits, some cost-sharing options, and a few specific additional service packages will be necessary to "keep competition focused on the twin dimensions of price and quality and not risk selection."
2. Define enrollment and marketing rules. The author calls for a one-year open-enrollment policy and careful supervision of consumer information by HCFA.
3. Collect and disseminate enough information to inform enrollees about comparative quality measures and to facilitate plan or provider switching. Nichols discusses the imperfect art of measuring medical outcomes and quality. He argues that effective competition depends on creating the incentives to learn how to make these measurements and to present them in a useful form to consumers.
4. Negotiate competitive bids with plans. The author argues that HCFA should use its large market share and market strength to obtain lower prices and accountability from competing plans.
5. Give consumers incentives to choose efficient plans. In what he calls the most complicated and controversial step, Nichols emphasizes the need to establish fixed government payment to give consumers an incentive to shop for efficient plans. He discusses the difficulty of establishing a fixed contribution based on a percentage of the lowest bid from competing plans and suggests a variation to overcome these difficulties.
6. Construct risk adjusters. Nichols discusses both the need for effective risk adjusters and the current state of knowledge for constructing them. He suggests several promising approaches for improving risk adjusters and calls for additional research.

Nichols concludes with the following cogent reminder: "A competitive health plan market can be the Medicare program's best long-run friend, but only if we structure the relationship carefully. We can do so, and the time to start is this afternoon. We will all be Medicare beneficiaries soon enough."

**At the Beginning.** H. E. Frech III laments that managed care dominates health policy discussions while traditional fee-for-service medicine dominates Medicare. He reminds us that managed care is only the tail in Medicare, while traditional FFS is the dog. Frech views traditional Medicare as the most promising starting place for reform. He reviews data on the movement to managed care in the private sector but argues that such a move would likely be slower in Medicare. As a consequence, traditional FFS will continue to dominate Medicare for the next several decades.

Frech traces the history of Medicare based on Blue Cross and Blue Shield plans of the mid-1960s and contrasts it with the private insurance market's change in benefit design and movement to managed care. He points out that both Medicare and tax policy have subsidized supplemental insurance (Medigap, as broadly defined); this process has raised the annual costs of the Medicare program by 20 percent, approximately $30 billion per year. To correct the basic problems with Medicare, he considers three broad areas for reform:

1. Prohibit or discourage supplemental insurance. To restore the cost-control features originally built into Medicare, Frech discusses several approaches designed to prohibit or change supplemental insurance: directly regulating Medigap policies; taxing Medigap policies; integrating Medicare and Medigap (by requiring Medigap policies to cover the entire range of Medicare benefits); and modernizing Medicare benefits to reduce the demand for supplemental insurance. These approaches are not mutually exclusive and might be combined to restore the cost-effective incentives expected with more cost-sharing and better catastrophic benefits.

2. Introduce options for expanded cost-sharing. Frech suggests that Medicare should offer beneficiaries more choices for more catastrophic benefits and more cost-sharing with policies that would meet their needs while reducing their demand for supplemental policies. This approach is not likely to be controversial for those with enough income to bear the risk, and the author suggests the use of medical savings accounts or retroactive rebates to provide for the lower-income sector.

3. Speed the transition to Medicare managed care. Frech points out that Medicare payment policies and regulations have fa-

vored traditional managed care of the health maintenance organization type (HMO) over less-structured forms, such as preferred provider organizations (PPOs) and point-of-service (POS) plans, which are likely to be more attractive to the elderly. He encourages the continuation of the changes included in the Balanced Budget Act to spur the more rapid development of these alternative forms of managed care.

**Competitive Pricing.** Targeting the bottom line, Bryan Dowd and Roger Feldman explain in chapter 7 that their proposal is designed to improve the efficiency of Medicare. They point out that Medicare faces "an intolerable problem of intergenerational fairness," which increased taxes are unlikely to solve. Their proposal sets the government's contribution as both a defined contribution and a defined benefit—a fixed payment across all plans that is based on the lowest-cost qualified health plan in each market area. Their rationale comes from their analysis of two ways to reduce the cost of Medicare: placing a limit on the government's contribution to Medicare premiums and creating incentives that induce beneficiaries to choose more cost-effective plans.

The authors point out that the terms *defined contribution* and *defined benefit*, borrowed from the terminology of employee pension plans, can be confusing when applied to multiple health plans and to Medicare. Although a defined contribution would promote both competition and budget control, it would not necessarily guarantee any level of Medicare benefits unless the contribution were somehow tied to the cost of providing those benefits. To achieve the twin objectives of improving efficiency and maintaining the value of the benefit, Dowd and Feldman propose that the government solicit bids from qualified health plans to deliver a specified level of benefits. The government's premium contribution would be based on the lowest bid for that package of benefits in each market area. By requiring the fee-for-service sector to participate in the bidding, the government would greatly improve its chances of establishing an undistorted price for the purchase of the set of benefits that it wishes to guarantee. The authors point out that because both consumer preferences (demand) and medical technology (supply) can change over time, their proposal would ensure that Medicare continues to purchase an efficient level of benefits over time.

Dowd and Feldman next address the difficult problem of risk selection, the fly-in-the-ointment argument in any discussion of efficiency in health markets. Even if the government did establish an efficient price through competitive bidding, does the choice by high-risk patients of the cost-effective plans or the cost-*in*effective plans threaten the system? The authors use a graphic model to illustrate why HCFA's requirement that plans use an average-cost community rating results in too few beneficiaries choosing cost-effective health plans. Dowd and Feldman conclude that efficiency would be improved if plans were allowed to charge beneficiaries their marginal cost for each plan. Such individual experience-rating may result in high-risk beneficiaries paying higher out-of-pocket premiums. That may be considered unfair, but it is more efficient.

According to the authors, empirical evidence shows that, on average, high-risk individuals prefer cost-*in*effective care. Dowd and Feldman analyze this situation and show that average-cost community rating without risk adjustment would produce an equilibrium in which primarily low-risk beneficiaries select cost-effective plans. This situation seems to occur when high-risk individuals forgo the extra benefits of managed care in order to stay in FFS.

Dowd and Feldman also analyze the role of information in promoting efficient consumer choice. They argue that if the government has better information about quality than beneficiaries do, providing that information to beneficiaries would improve the efficiency of their choices. They doubt that the government can use information more efficiently than individuals.

**FEHBP as a Model.** Walton Francis, for nineteen years the author of *Checkbook*'s annual comparison of health plans, examines the use of the Federal Employees Health Benefits Program (FEHBP) as a model for Medicare reform. He reviews the present operation of the FEHBP and compares its performance with that of Medicare over the past two decades. The author argues that the FEHBP has dramatically outperformed Medicare with lower cost increases, modernization of benefits, and more efficient administration. In highlighting risk selection, Francis distinguishes between desirable risk selection, which reflects consumers' preferences, and destructive risk selection, which leads to market failure in insurance markets. While some FEHBP plans have failed, destructive risk selection rarely occurs, and the program has remained remarkably stable despite having few tools to deal with risk selection. The political nature of changes to Medicare contrasts strongly with the relative efficiency of FEHBP's adjustment to change.

The author analyzes both the opportunities and the pitfalls of the FEHBP as a model for Medicare reform. In reviewing the potential of Medicare+Choice established in the Balanced Budget Act of 1997, he reminds us—as do the other authors in this volume—that establishing a competitive market under existing law is problematic as long as traditional fee-for-service Medicare remains dominant. In discussing the major policy dilemmas in Medicare reform, he presents several practical solutions. The following examples illustrate the nature of these suggestions.

- If Medicare contributions were tied to benefit costs, there is concern that Congress or the administration would have strong incentives either to reduce benefits to save costs or to raise out-of-pocket payments by enrollees. To avoid this problem, Francis suggests that annual contributions be based on a rolling average of benefit costs. This change would allow plans to adjust to changing consumer demands without a major effect on either the next budget or payments by enrollees.
- To protect Medicare recipients against the loss of benefits now guaranteed under current law, while allowing plans to compete on the basis of benefit design (a major advantage of the FEHBP), Francis suggests that benefits be tied to actuarial measures of performance. This practice is similar to those now used in the FEHBP program.
- To help manage risk selection, the author proposes a reinsurance system that would make retrospective adjustments to federal contributions based on the actual distribution of high-cost cases. Such a system would be especially important to small plans and would help alleviate the problems with inaccurate estimates of plan costs.
- To protect traditional Medicare against adverse selection, Francis suggests that Medicare's administrative agency be given some latitude to change benefits, cost sharing, and geographic premiums in traditional Medicare to compete with choice plans. A major advantage of the FEHBP over Medicare has been its ability to make small changes in the program without congressional consideration.

A central theme in chapter 8 is the FEHBP's outperformance of Medicare because it could take advantage of competition and consumer choice. The FEHBP is not a perfect system, but, unlike Medicare, it has had the flexibility to respond to its problems. The principal lesson from the FEHBP's experience is that a perfect plan for Medicare reform may not be possible. But we can design a new Medicare program that is fair to beneficiaries, is more efficient than the current program, and has the ability to solve future problems.

## Conclusion

If we look at the history of Medicare, especially the twenty years of contentious political debates preceding its passage in 1965, the highly political nature of today's debate on reform should not surprise anyone (Helms 1999). The economists who have contributed the essays in this volume can do little to calm the political waters surrounding Medicare. Our modest objective is to stress that to the extent we can improve the efficiency of the program, more resources will be available to improve the fairness of the program. As Len Nichols writes, the time to start seeking fair and efficient reform is this afternoon.

## Notes

1. Much of the economic literature predicts that when price controls create shortages, nonprice discrimination on the part of providers will increase. Each provider would choose to allocate available time among all those seeking services according to the individual provider's preferences, including the willingness to provide free care and to treat difficult medical conditions. If some physicians chose not to treat some Medicare patients, the remaining physicians not wishing to discriminate would encounter increasing difficulty in caring for additional Medicare patients.

2. Contributions include the employee's and employer's share of HI payroll taxes, interest, and SMI premiums. Values are discounted with the average interest rate on the HI trust fund over the same period (Committee on Ways and Means 1998, 126).

3. There is a time dimension to economic efficiency, because making any market change too quickly or too slowly may be wasteful. In medical markets, the efficient introduction of new technologies may be affected by the desire of consumers and producers to determine the relative effectiveness and safety of each innovation.

# References

Auerbach, Alan J., Jagadeesh Gokhale, and Laurence J. Kotlikoff. 1991. "Generational Accounts: A Meaningful Alternative to Deficit Accounting." In *Tax Policy and the Economy*, edited by David Bradford, vol. 5, pp. 55–110. Cambridge: MIT Press.

Board of Trustees of the Federal Hospital Insurance Trust Fund. 1999. *1999 Annual Report of the Board of Trustees of the Federal Hospital Insurance Trust Fund.* Washington, D.C.: Government Printing Office.

Board of Trustees of the Federal Supplementary Medical Insurance Trust Fund. 1999. *1999 Annual Report of the Board of Trustees of the Supplementary Medical Insurance Trust Fund,* pp. 2–3. Washington, D.C.: Government Printing Office.

Congressional Budget Office. 1997. *Budgetary Implications of the Balanced Budget Act of 1997.* Washington, D.C.: Congressional Budget Office.

———. 1998a. *The Economic and Budget Outlook: Fiscal Years 1999–2008,* pp. 63–79. Washington, D.C.: Government Printing Office.

———. 1998b. *Long-Term Budgetary Pressures and Policy Options,* p. xvi. Washington, D.C.: Government Printing Office.

Dowd, Bryan. 1999. "An Unusual View of Health Economics." *Health Affairs* 18 (1) (January–February): 266–69.

Gaynor, Martin, and William Vogt. 1997."What Does Economics Have to Say about Health Policy, Anyway? A Comment on Evans and Rice." *Journal of Health Politics, Policy and Law* 22 (2) (April): 475–96.

Gokhale, Jagadeesh, and Laurence J. Kotlikoff. 1998. *Medicare from the Perspective of Generational Accounting.* National Bureau of Economic Research Working Paper 6596. Washington, D.C.

Helms, Robert B. 1999. "The Origins of Medicare." *The World & I* 14 (3) (March): 40–45.

Kahn, Charles N., III, and Hans Kuttner. 1999. "Budget Bills and Medicare Policy: The Politics of the BBA." *Health Affairs* 18 (1) (January–February): 37–47.

Kaiser Family Foundation. 1998. "National Survey on Medicare: The Next Big Health Policy Debate?" www.kff.org, chart 10.

Kaiser Family Foundation–Harvard University. 1999. "Post-Election Survey: Priorities for the 106th Congress," www.kff.org, question 1.

King, Roland. 1996. "The New Medicare Trust Fund Report." American Enterprise Institute. Washington, D.C.

Kotlikoff, Laurence J. 1992. *Generational Accounting*. New York: Free Press.

Moon, Marilyn. 1997. "Restructuring Medicare's Cost-Sharing." Paper presented at National Academy of Social Insurance Study Panel on Medicare's Long-Term Financing, table 2. Washington, D.C.

———. 1999. "Will the Care Be There? Vulnerable Beneficiaries and Medicare Reform." *Health Affairs* 18 (1) (January–February): 107–17.

National Bipartisan Commission on the Future of Medicare. 1998. *Income and Assets of the Elderly and Near Elderly*. Washington, D.C. See http://thomas.loc.gov/medicare/dowdall.html.

Pauly, Mark. 1997. "Who Was That Straw Man Anyway? A Comment on Evans and Rice." *Journal of Health Politics, Policy and Law* 22 (2) (April): 467–73.

Peterson, Peter G. 1996. *Will America Grow Up Before It Grows Old? How the Coming Social Security Crisis Threatens You, Your Family, and Your Country*. New York: Random House.

Reischauer, Robert D. 1997. "Medicare: Beyond 2002." In *Policy Options for Reforming the Medicare Program*, edited by Stuart H. Altman, Uwe Reinhardt, and David Shactman. Princeton: Robert Wood Johnson Foundation.

Rice, Thomas. 1998. *The Economics of Health Reconsidered*. Chicago: Health Administration Press.

Robertson, A. Haeworth. 1997. *The Big Lie: What Every Baby Boomer Should Know about Social Security and Medicare*. Washington, D.C.: Retirement Policy Institute.

Smith, Adam. 1937. *The Wealth of Nations*, p. 423. New York: Modern Library.

U.S. Bureau of the Census. 1997. *1997 Statistical Abstract of the United States*, p. 122. Washington, D.C.: Government Printing Office.

U.S. Department of Health and Human Services, Health Care Financing Administration. 1998. *The Profiles of Medicare: Chart Book*. Washington, D.C.: Government Printing Office.

U.S. House of Representatives, Committee on Ways and Means. 1998. *1998 Green Book*. Washington, D.C.: Government Printing Office.

Weaver, Carolyn L. Forthcoming. *Social Security and Its Reform*. Washington, D.C.: AEI Press.

Weicher, John C. 1995. "The Distribution of Wealth: Increasing Inequality?" *Federal Reserve Bank of St. Louis Review* 77 (1) (January–February): 5–23.

————. 1997. "Wealth and Its Distribution, 1983–1992: Secular Growth, Cyclical Stability." *Federal Reserve Bank of St. Louis Review* 79 (2) (January–February): 3–19.

Wilensky, Gail R., and Joseph P. Newhouse. 1999. "Medicare: What's Right? What's Wrong? What's Next?" *Health Affairs* 18 (1) (January–February): 92–106.

# 2

# The Bumpy Road to Reform

## Joseph R. Antos and Linda Bilheimer

The rapid growth of Medicare spending has been a continuing concern of policymakers since the program's creation in 1965. Between 1978 and 1998, mandatory Medicare outlays—rising from 1.1 percent to 2.5 percent of the gross domestic product—grew at an average rate of more than 11 percent a year. The program has absorbed an expanding share of the goods and services produced in this country and is now the second largest federal program, after Social Security. Medicare will spend about $216 billion, about 13 percent of federal outlays, in 1999.

Nonetheless, Medicare expenditures barely grew in 1998. But that slowdown, continuing in 1999, reflects short-term responses to recent legislative and regulatory changes and not a permanent reduction in spending growth. Little has changed to affect the tremendous financial pressures that the program will be placing on the federal budget—pressures resulting from the baby boomers aging into the program and from the rising health care costs per beneficiary.

---

The views expressed here are those of the authors and do not necessarily represent the views of the Congressional Budget Office.

The public seems unready to acknowledge that Medicare needs substantial reforms if it is to be preserved for future generations. Many people still believe that their payroll taxes are paying for their own future benefits, rather than the benefits of current enrollees. That perception has established a strong sense of entitlement that hinders consideration of unpopular policy options. Through polls and focus groups, people indicate that they do not want to pay higher taxes to support the program or pay significantly more for services. Nor do they want to reduce payments for providers or raise the age of eligibility for benefits. Meanwhile, the beneficiaries' demand for coverage of prescription drugs is growing. Offering prescription drugs would greatly improve the program's benefits but also raise its costs substantially.

Many Medicare beneficiaries believe that fraud by providers is the main cause of rising program costs; they argue that the primary policy focus should be reducing program fraud and abuse. Initiatives for reducing fraud and abuse may, indeed, decrease spending growth in the short term and are important for preserving program integrity. But such initiatives will do little to change Medicare's long-term cost trends. More fundamental restructuring is required to put the program on the road to long-term financial stability.

This chapter examines strategies for reforming Medicare. It first considers the sources of rapid growth in spending over the long term and discusses design aspects of the program that contribute to inefficiency. It then reviews several options for reforming the program and discusses future directions.

## Long-Term Cost and Financing

Analysts have long recognized that the aging of the baby boomers will place unprecedented demands on Medicare, if only because of the large number of beneficiaries added to the program. Based on the intermediate assumptions of the Social Security trustees, the elderly population will grow by slightly more than 1 percent a year between 2000 and 2010, the year in which the baby boomers begin to retire. Between 2010 and 2030, the elderly population will grow at an annual rate of almost 3 percent, from 39 million to 69 million. Because of increased longevity, the proportion of that population that will be older than seventy-five will rise as well.

Medicare costs are likely to grow much faster than program enrollment, however. The cost per beneficiary of providing health care services, which has risen dramatically, is likely to continue to grow rapidly. That growth reflects both advances in medical technology that will raise health care costs and continuing increases in the beneficiaries' use of services.

Medicare spending is projected to rise from about 2.5 percent of GDP in 1998 to 6.3 percent in 2030, as the last of the boomers enroll in the program.[1] But that projection, which is based on methods used by Medicare's trustees, is optimistic. It assumes that growth in Medicare spending per beneficiary will gradually decline to be more in line with the growth in hourly earnings, even without a significant policy change. Consequently, after 2020, the projected growth in Medicare spending as a share of GDP accounts only for the growth in the number of Medicare beneficiaries as a share of the population. That assumption may be unrealistic: if spending per beneficiary does not slow, Medicare's share of GDP would be significantly higher.

Meanwhile, the proportion of active workers to elderly people will fall and will make the current financing system difficult to maintain without tax increases or substantial cost reductions. In 1998 the United States had 3.9 workers per Medicare beneficiary; by 2030 it will have only 2.3 workers per beneficiary.[2]

Those stark facts make a strong case for reform. But the idiosyncrasies of Medicare's financing, and confusion about the meaning of trust fund financing, often obfuscate the policy debate. Medicare operates on a pay-as-you-go basis financed through payroll taxes and through general revenues, with beneficiaries paying a modest premium that covers about 10 percent of the total cost of the program. The hospital insurance (HI) trust fund, which pays for inpatient hospital services and postacute care, is financed primarily by the payroll tax. Since that trust fund's revenues are limited, it can become depleted if outlays exceed income over time. The Congressional Budget Office projects that HI trust fund outlays will exceed income by 2007 and the fund will become technically insolvent some years after 2010.

In contrast to the HI trust fund, the supplementary medical insurance (SMI) trust fund, which pays for physician and other ambulatory medical services, is financed with general revenues and premiums paid by beneficiaries. Since general revenue financing is not capped, the SMI trust fund cannot be depleted. But because SMI outlays are likely to continue growing faster than either general revenues or premiums, SMI is no more financially sound than HI.

Some policies to delay the insolvency of the HI trust fund, such as changing how Medicare pays for postacute services, may slow spending growth. But other policies, such as boosting trust fund revenues or switching the financing of services from HI to SMI (which happened with some home health services as a result of the Balanced Budget Act of 1997), improve the fund's financial status without addressing the underlying growth in costs. Indeed, depleting the HI trust fund could be avoided indefinitely by transferring general revenues to it as necessary, as now occurs with the SMI trust fund. Although the latest projections of HI trust fund balances sway the public perception of Medicare's financial health, those projections can shift significantly from year to year without any real change in Medicare's long-term financial status.

## Problems with Medicare's Design

In important respects, Medicare has become an archaic and dysfunctional program. Several of the program's main features provide inappropriate incentives for the use of health services, helping to increase program costs without substantially improving the health status of beneficiaries. Significant obstacles to Medicare's fiscal stability include

- the dominance of traditional fee-for-service Medicare;
- the prevalence of insurance supplements that blunt beneficiaries' cost-consciousness;
- the lack of price competition among Medicare managed-care plans; and
- inadequate regulatory payment methods.

Medicare operates in a largely unmanaged fee-for-service environment, which is rapidly disappearing from the larger private health care market. Although most Medicare enrollees may enroll in a managed-care plan, a large majority—about 84 percent in 1999—have chosen to remain in the traditional fee-for-service sector, with its open-ended claims on federal payments. Fee-for-service arrangements encourage providers to supply covered services. Although fee-for-service enrollees face considerable cost-sharing requirements, which might otherwise dampen their demand for services, most of them have supplemental coverage that pays some or all of their deductibles and coinsurance.

In 1996, for example, about two-thirds of Medicare fee-for-service enrollees had private supplemental insurance, and an additional 15 percent had Medicaid coverage for their deductibles and coinsurance (Eppig and Chulis 1997). Enrollees with private supplements were about evenly divided between those with employer-sponsored plans and those with individual Medigap policies that they purchased themselves. (A small percentage had both types of private supplemental coverage.) Fee-for-service enrollees with Medicaid coverage, and many of those with Medigap plans, have full first-dollar coverage, so they have no financial incentive to curb their use of covered Medicare services. By contrast, those enrollees with supplements from their former employers are less likely to have coverage for all their Medicare cost sharing; employer-sponsored supplemental plans typically reduce but do not eliminate cost-sharing requirements.

Differences in supplemental coverage among fee-for-service enrollees result in marked differences in their use of Medicare services. Christensen and Shinogle (1997) estimated that fee-for-service enrollees with Medigap plans used 28 percent more services than enrollees with no supplement, and enrollees with employer-sponsored supplements used 17 percent more services than those with no supplement. The additional demand for Medicare services that resulted from supplemental coverage raised program expenditures in 1998 by as much as $17 billion.

In contrast to fee-for-service providers, managed-care plans have incentives to constrain the use of services, because the plans are financially responsible for the services that they provide. But because of defects in payment and enrollment policies, Medicare's managed-care plans contribute little to program savings. Medicare ties its payments to health maintenance organizations to costs in the fee-for-service sector. Consequently, the program does not capture savings from more efficient health plans. Furthermore, if an HMO makes higher profits under Medicare than in its private business, the excess profits must be returned as additional benefits.[3] Thus, managed care has resulted in more benefits for enrollees rather than lower costs for Medicare.

In addition, Medicare overpays HMOs on average because of favorable selection: beneficiaries who enroll in HMOs use fewer services on average than beneficiaries who remain in traditional Medicare. Favorable selection may result from sicker patients wishing to continue to have access to their personal physicians and not wanting constraints on their choice of specialists. Some frail elderly beneficiaries may also choose to stay in the fee-for-service sector because of the open-ended home health benefits offered. HMOs that offer generous prescription drug benefits, however, may attract less-healthy enrollees.

Prior to the Balanced Budget Act, Medicare's enrollment rules encouraged favorable selection into managed-care plans; beneficiaries could change plans with little restriction and move freely between the managed-care and fee-for-service sectors. Beneficiaries who enrolled in managed-care plans when they were relatively healthy could easily transfer back into fee-for-service if they became ill or dissatisfied with the specialist services that their plan offered. (The only disincentive to returning to traditional Medicare under those circumstances was the potential difficulty of obtaining Medigap coverage at an affordable premium.) That flexibility will be reduced as a result of the budget act, which is phasing in some restrictions on the ability of beneficiaries to change plans.

In principle, Medicare can adjust its payments to managed-care plans to reflect enrollees' health risks. But risk-adjustment methods are still rudimentary, and the adjusters that Medicare uses explain only about 1 percent of the variation in actual spending. Before the Balanced Budget Act, inadequate risk-adjustment resulted in an 8 percent overpayment to Medicare risk plans, on average (Riley et al. 1996). Payment reductions instituted by the BBA would largely eliminate the excess payment over the next few years, but those general reductions in payments may not be closely related to the variation in costs that individual plans incur. Hence, the main effect of those reductions could be to underpay some plans (which would probably cut benefits or drop out of Medicare+Choice), while continuing to overpay other plans.

## Policy Options

Policymakers have developed many proposals, ranging from relatively simple adjustments in the program to full-scale restructuring, to address Medicare's long-term financing crisis. Broadly speaking, three types of options have been proposed:

- Options that reduce program costs without improving its efficiency. Examples of such options include controlling prices paid to providers, placing limits on covered services, and increasing the age of Medicare eligibility. Such options might be part of a larger reform proposal, but they are insufficient by themselves to ensure the program's financial stability.
- Options that would reduce costs and improve efficiency. Some of those options would make improvements within Medicare's current structure, particularly regarding how the fee-for-service

program operates. Others, such as voucher proposals, would restructure Medicare into a competitive marketplace.

- Options that would restructure Medicare's financing. Proposals to convert Medicare from pay-as-you-go to prefunding address the inappropriate incentives of the current financing system.

Other options, which would increase program revenues by raising premiums or taxes without making other changes, do not address the fundamental issues facing Medicare and are not discussed here.

**Reducing Costs without Improving Efficiency.** Efforts to constrain the growth of Medicare spending have traditionally focused on limiting the growth in the price of services. Payment rates for hospital and physician services, for example, are updated periodically to reflect inflation and increases in input costs. But those updates have often been reduced through legislation. Such policies seem to place the burden of cost containment on providers, who presumably have deeper pockets than beneficiaries.

However, limiting the growth of prices in the fee-for-service sector does nothing to change the incentive of providers to offer more services. Thus, such policies may not effectively curb spending growth, which depends on both prices and quantities of services used. Moreover, if payment rates are severely constrained, providers may drop out of Medicare or limit the types of services provided to beneficiaries or the number of Medicare patients whom they will treat.

The counterpart to limiting the price of services is limiting the use of those services, for example, either by not covering certain services at all or by paying for only a limited number of days of care. Medicare generally covers all services deemed medically necessary without restricting their use, and limits on benefits are clearly unpopular with beneficiaries and policymakers.

An alternative approach to reducing benefits would raise the age of Medicare eligibility from sixty-five to sixty-seven. The delay in eligibility could be phased in over several years, much as the retirement age for Social Security is being raised to age sixty-seven by 2025. Compared with current law, that option would reduce Medicare enrollment by about 7 percent and spending by about 3 percent a year once it was fully phased in (CBO 1998b, 52).

But such a policy would shift costs that are now paid by Medicare to individuals and employers who continued to offer health insurance to their retirees. Higher costs to employers would likely reduce the number that offered retiree health benefits. Allowing otherwise ineligible people older than sixty-two or sixty-five to buy into Medicare would alleviate that problem. The cost of a buy-in would be substantial, however, perhaps as much as $4,800 in the year 2000 for each person enrolled (CBO 1998a, 39). A subsidized buy-in would be more accessible to low- and middle-income people, but the subsidy would increase the costs of Medicare.

**Reducing Costs and Improving Program Efficiency.** Various policies have been developed in recent years to offer incentives for both providers and beneficiaries to use health care resources more efficiently. Many of those options would improve the operation of the fee-for-service sector without significantly restructuring the overall program. Because fee-for-service Medicare is likely to remain the largest part of the program for many years, improving its operation could yield substantial savings. Improving the efficiency of the traditional program is also important if that program is to survive in the long term under a more competitive system. Creating such a system, which would enable beneficiaries to choose from an array of competing health plans, is the objective of voucher proposals.

**Payment Methods and Management Tools.** Medicare has instituted a number of administrative mechanisms designed to improve providers' efficiency. Prospective payment systems (PPSs), for instance, provide incentives to reduce the costs of treatment. Other management tools used by private health plans could be adopted to improve providers' efficiency.

Paying separately for the individual components of a patient's treatment encourages the use of unnecessary services. In contrast, a single predetermined payment covering a set of related services discourages the overuse of services. Thus, the PPS for inpatient hospital services pays a fixed amount for most services furnished during an inpatient stay. Hospitals try to minimize their costs for providing a combined set of services by eliminating duplication and shortening lengths of stay. Efforts are under way to develop similar systems for other services, including those delivered through hospital outpatient departments, skilled nursing facilities, and home health agencies.

That concept could be applied more comprehensively. Hospital PPS payments could be broadened to incorporate both hospital services and physician services rendered during an inpatient stay. That payment method has been successfully tested in a recent demonstration project focusing on heart bypass operations (Cromwell et al. 1997). Similarly, hospital PPS payments could be expanded to include postacute care provided by skilled nursing facilities and home health agencies. Bundling payments across inpatient and postacute settings for diagnoses with a significant postacute care component could result in a more efficient allocation of resources.

True prospective payment systems are difficult to develop, however. The services included in the payment bundle must be closely related to each other from a clinical perspective. Broader bundles that more fully encompass the care needed to treat a patient provide more opportunity for increasing efficiency but impose greater financial risks on providers. Payment adjustments to reflect the severity of different patients' conditions are needed to ensure that the prospective payment is appropriate and does not discourage providers from treating difficult cases.

In addition to improving Medicare payment systems, other tools would enhance management of the program. Competitive bidding, for example, might be used in place of administered pricing to set payment levels. Bidding models to set the prices of clinical laboratory and other services have already been developed, and the Health Care Financing Administration is proposing to test a market-based pricing system to set HMO payments in Phoenix and Kansas City, but is facing local resistance from the managed-care industry. Negotiated pricing was successfully tested in the heart bypass demonstration, as mentioned. Private health plans use selective contracting, physician profiling, and preferred provider arrangements, all of which could help to reduce costs in fee-for-service Medicare.

**Cost-Sharing Strategies and Limits on Supplementary Coverage.** Medicare's cost-sharing requirements are a complicated system of deductibles and coinsurance rates that vary by service. Unlike most other health insurance policies, Medicare has separate deductibles for hospital and physician services. Moreover, the program does not limit the beneficiaries' out-of-pocket liability. Recent proposals would simplify those requirements to a single deductible and a uniform coinsurance rate for all covered services and would cap beneficiaries' total liability.

Some proposals would also limit the role of supplementary insurance. If annual out-of-pocket costs were capped and supplementary insurance prohibited from offering first-dollar coverage, beneficiaries would have less reason to seek those supplements. Beneficiaries would also use somewhat fewer covered services, given their increased direct liability for the costs. Such a proposal could yield substantial program savings.

An ambitious proposal to revamp cost-sharing requirements and limit the scope of supplementary coverage would face major obstacles, however. The increased federal regulation of insurance, particularly the regulation of employer-sponsored retiree plans, could be problematic. Rather than try to limit coverage in such plans—which would be an unprecedented step—some analysts have suggested taxing enrollees with private supplemental coverage. The tax would be equivalent to the average cost of the additional Medicare services induced by first-dollar coverage.

**Vouchers.** Voucher proposals shift the focus of payment from providers to beneficiaries. Beneficiaries choose among competing health plans; market forces determine the premiums. The federal contribution is limited, however, and beneficiaries selecting plans with premiums costing more than the federal contribution would be required to pay the difference. Such proposals seek to enhance the beneficiaries' cost-consciousness regarding their choice of health plan rather than to delay such considerations until they face treatment decisions. In principle, health plans would compete on price and benefits and would have incentives to improve efficiency, to lower their costs, and thus to increase their market share.

Proposals for vouchers differ considerably regarding limits on the federal contribution and the requirements for health plans competing for Medicare business. Vouchers are not synonymous with defined-contribution plans. Pure defined-contribution plans fix the amount of the federal contribution to premiums without specifying a basic set of mandatory benefits. Such an option would shift the financial risk of rising health care costs from the federal government to Medicare beneficiaries, unless the federal payment grew as rapidly as those costs.

Other voucher proposals would allow the federal contribution to vary according to the premium charged by the health plan and might impose some restrictions on the benefits offered by competing plans. The Federal Employees Health Benefits Program (FEHBP) is the best-known example of a voucher plan. Benefits are not standardized, but the Office of Personnel Management approves any benefit changes. The plans and OPM negotiate premiums. The maximum federal contribution equals 72 percent of the average premium for all plans, and employees pay at least 25 percent of the premium for the plan that they choose. In 1997, for example, the federal contribution for individuals ranged from about $1,000 to $1,600, and individuals contributed from about $400 to $1,800 for a year's coverage (NASI 1998, 29).

Another alternative, dubbed the premium support model, would require all plans to cover a core set of benefits. Plans could offer additional services and set higher premiums, but the basic benefits would have to be priced separately to facilitate comparison shopping by beneficiaries. The government's payment would ensure that beneficiaries could buy at least one plan and pay no more than a modest premium. Policymakers would determine the basic benefit package and, in particular, whether the package should include prescription drugs.

The growth of Medicare outlays under a voucher proposal would depend on how health plans competed in that market. If the government's premium contribution were adjusted to reflect more accurately the expected costs of providing services to individual beneficiaries, risk selection would be reduced, and competition among plans would be more effective. Plans that attracted disproportionate numbers of high-cost enrollees would find it difficult to compete if the payments that they could expect for those people did not reflect the plans' probable costs. Instead of focusing on improving efficiency, plans under those circumstances might focus on attracting healthier enrollees.

Risk adjustment is still a primitive science, however, and the data requirements for the most promising risk-adjustment systems exceed what many health plans can now provide. Less complex adjusters that depend only on partial information about the patient's use of services might feasibly be implemented relatively quickly. But adjusters based on readily available data, such as inpatient hospitalization rates, would reward plans for treating patients in hospitals rather than in other, possibly more cost-effective, settings.

Other strategies could, however, limit the extent to which plans face adverse selection in enrollment. The use of coordinated open-enrollment periods, for example, would provide all beneficiaries the opportunity to choose plans on an equal basis. Moreover, if beneficiaries could switch plans only once a year during the open-enrollment period, they would be less likely to shift between managed-care and fee-for-service Medicare as their health status changed. In addition, the marketing practices of health plans might be restricted to reduce the opportunities to target preferred beneficiaries. Requiring plans to offer a standardized benefit package would prevent plans from tailoring their benefits to attract healthier beneficiaries. Such a requirement, however, would force some beneficiaries to accept plans offering greater or fewer benefits than they would have chosen in an unrestricted market.

Adjusting federal payments for health risks is only part of the price-setting process required by a voucher system. In addition, a method to establish each plan's total premium must be implemented to foster competition and keep the growth of premiums in check.

Competitive bidding approaches might be feasible in some markets, but comparing the prices of health plans offering different benefits would be difficult. Requiring a standard set of core benefits would simplify such comparisons and would encourage price competition among plans. Any additional benefits offered by plans could be priced separately. In markets that are too small to support more than one or two plans, negotiations with health plans could establish realistic premiums. The experience of FEHBP, moreover, suggests that negotiations for premiums, benefits, or other conditions of participation in Medicare might be a useful adjunct to competitive bidding. If, for example, the Medicare regulatory authority thought that all bids in a market were too high, jawboning might lower them.

In addition to determining how to establish premiums under a voucher system, policymakers would need to set the federal government's contribution toward premiums and the growth of that contribution over time. The government contribution might be reduced for beneficiaries with higher incomes, although that policy might be difficult to administer. Limiting the growth in the average contribution poses more substantive concerns. A cap on the annual growth in the government's average contribution per beneficiary would safeguard the Treasury from excessive cost increases and discourage plans from allowing their costs to rise too rapidly. Such a cap, however, would shift some of the risk of rising health costs to beneficiaries, who would have only a limited ability to avoid those costs by enrolling in lower-cost plans.

A voucher-style system would be less likely to succeed if the traditional fee-for-service program did not become a fully competitive plan within the system and did not operate on the same basis as all other plans. To compete successfully, fee-for-service Medicare would need the authority to use the same tools used by other plans to manage costs aggressively. And it would have to be held accountable for its management of costs. The growth of Medicare spending as a share of national income could not be reduced if the plan with the largest enrollment continued to need substantial subsidies from general revenues.

**Restructuring Medicare's Financing.** Voucher proposals have typically emphasized the importance of vigorous competition among health plans to ensure efficiency and maintain high standards of quality in the health care provided by the plans. Those proposals, however, generally do not address changes in Medicare's financing. Recently some analysts have suggested that replacing Medicare's pay-as-you-go financing scheme with a prefunded system would promote both health plan competition and beneficiary choice.

Proposals to prefund Medicare would require people to save during their working years to finance health insurance after they retire. Ironically, this approach would establish a self-financing mechanism that many people believe the Medicare trust funds already provide. Prefunding is designed to eliminate the flow of subsidies from workers to retirees. Those subsidies will become increasingly burdensome under the current Medicare system, as the number of workers for each retiree falls over the next several decades. Unlike pay-as-you-go financing, prefunding intends to tap the aggregate lifetime income of a cohort to pay fully for the aggregate health expenditures of that cohort when it retires.

Two approaches have been proposed to prefund health insurance needs in retirement. The first approach would require people to invest in medical retirement accounts (MRAs) that could be used to purchase insurance in the individual market at retirement. MRA funds might also pay for health expenses not covered by insurance. Contributions to the accounts and earnings from the investments could receive favorable tax treatment.

The second approach would require young people to purchase health plans that would guarantee coverage at retirement. This approach would reduce the risk that people who become medically uninsurable before retirement could not find coverage. Unfortunately, the health plan purchased by a person in his twenties might no longer be appropriate or might no longer exist forty years later. Alternatively, insurers and health plans might be required to guarantee coverage to those reaching age sixty-five regardless of their medical condition. Risk-pooling arrangements could spread the costs of coverage for those people among all health plans.

Most prefunding proposals assume that retirees would choose whatever type of plan they wanted, with market forces determining premiums and covered benefits. In that environment, health plans would have incentives to compete on the basis of both price and quality, as well as covered benefits—incentives that Medicare lacks today.

To avoid free-rider problems, participation in a prefunded system would be mandatory. Not everyone could make contributions sufficient to finance even minimal insurance, however. If universal coverage for the elderly, a hallmark of the current Medicare program, were to be maintained, redistributing resources to the poor would continue to be necessary, although such redistribution might fall outside Medicare.

Prefunding would give individuals an ownership right to their health care benefits and would encourage price sensitivity in purchasing health care. But that system would shift more of the financial risk of health expenditures for the elderly from the federal government to individuals, in a change that would be politically controversial.

Prefunding also raises the issue of investment risk. If individuals depleted their MRA funds because of bad investments or poor timing, they would presumably be eligible for some federal health insurance subsidy. A reasonably generous subsidy might encourage people to make overly speculative investments. Thus, policymakers would have to decide how much government regulation of investment options would be necessary to balance financial risks and rates of return on investment.

Any switch from a pay-as-you-go system to prefunding would impose a major financial burden on individuals in the transition cohort. Those enrolled in Medicare during the transition and older workers who have insufficient working years left to save enough to cover their health costs in retirement would continue to depend on pay-as-you-go financing. Younger workers would face significant mandatory contributions to finance their own future insurance needs, while paying additional taxes to fund the transition.

Many discussions on the prefunding of Medicare focus on the macroeconomic effects of such proposals on the saving rate and, consequently, on the growth rate of the economy. If prefunding raised the net saving rate, it would enhance the long-term ability of the economy to provide health care and other goods and services. But how much of the required savings in MRAs would represent net additional savings is unclear. Those discussions often understate the importance of developing a competitive market for Medicare that offers strong financial incentives to improve the program's efficiency. Finding a better way to raise revenues, even one that provides a significant spur to the economy, could fail to resolve the larger policy problem unless the growth of Medicare spending is slowed.

# Road to Reform?

Policymakers seem to agree that Medicare needs reform, but they disagree on what the reform might be. There are many options; most are difficult to implement and politically unpalatable. The situation might be a recipe for stalemate. Despite substantial disagreements among policymakers on the direction of change, however, the Balanced Budget Act of 1997 took some halting steps toward reform.

**The Balanced Budget Act of 1997.** The Balanced Budget Act of 1997 included provisions to slow the short-term growth of Medicare spending and to pave the way for more fundamental, long-term restructuring of the program. The act had two important goals: to improve the efficiency of Medicare's fee-for-service system through payment reforms and to lay the groundwork for a more competitive system through the creation of the Medicare+Choice program. Although some provisions in the budget act represent potentially significant reforms, it is unclear whether those provisions can be implemented successfully. More fundamentally, the act did not address some of Medicare's underlying structural problems and therefore may not lead the Medicare program toward long-term financial stability.

The act's major fee-for-service reforms focused on establishing prospective payment systems for several major services that had been paid on the basis of their costs, including outpatient hospital services, skilled nursing facility services, and home health care. Prospective payment systems are extraordinarily difficult to design, however, in part because of the complexity of developing adequate risk-adjustment mechanisms, as discussed. Because of those difficulties, the new prospective payment mechanisms will probably resemble administratively determined fee schedules and may fail to blunt the incentives of current payment methods to expand the volume of patient services.

With home health care, for example, payments are likely to be based on a fixed amount per day rather than per episode of care. Such an approach would encourage home health agencies to limit the amount of services provided per day and to increase the number of days of care, and thus have an uncertain impact on program costs. Because of that potential outcome, the Medicare Payment Advisory Commission recently recommended that Congress impose modest cost-sharing requirements for home health services to dampen demand (Medicare Payment Advisory Commission 1999, 94).

In addition, the budget act established the Medicare + Choice program to expand managed-care options for beneficiaries, to attract more enrollees to managed care, and to foster competition among plans. To limit favorable selection into managed-care plans, the law requires HCFA to develop a risk-adjustment mechanism that reflects the health status of enrollees and to phase in restrictions on the ability of beneficiaries to switch plans.

Those provisions represent important steps toward a more competitive marketplace. Nonetheless, how plans will compete on the basis of price is not wholly clear. Medicare's payments to plans are still based on administered prices linked to the fee-for-service system. And the program continues its bias toward adding optional benefits rather than reducing the premium for the basic benefit package. More fundamentally, the traditional fee-for-service system, in which most beneficiaries participate, remains outside the competitive market.

The first year of implementation for Medicare + Choice has not been smooth. Complex changes in payment policy and new regulatory requirements demand substantial efforts by both health plans and HCFA. Moreover, the budget act imposed tight constraints on the growth of aggregate payments to managed-care plans through 2002, and some payments were reallocated from high-cost to low-cost areas. Some Medicare plans, therefore, were stunned by the small payment increases in 1998, as they were grappling with the new regulatory requirements.

Only three non-HMO plans applied to participate in Medicare + Choice in 1999. Forty-two HMO contractors, with some 420,000 beneficiaries, dropped out of the program. Those developments may not be significant, however. The exodus represents only one year's growth in the number of plans participating in the program. Moreover, Medicare risk plans are available in more counties now than in 1997.

**Future Direction of Reform.** The enormous popularity of Medicare and its fee-for-service sector poses the biggest obstacle to its reform. But preserving the program without change is unrealistic. That conclusion does not imply that Medicare's share of national income should not increase in the coming decades. The nation's ability to pay for health care grows as the economy grows, and that spending share could increase to some extent without adverse consequences. Moreover, since the elderly will become an increasingly dominant group in society, public acceptance of higher health expenditures will probably grow. But the trade-offs between health care and other goods and services would be less marked if Medicare were more efficient, so that enrollees' needs were met in the least costly way and demands for health care reflected the true costs and benefits of that care. Movement toward that goal requires the adoption of proposals to restructure Medicare.

The sheer variety of policy options is breathtaking, but certain themes emerge. Some options offer short-term fixes; others provide longer-term incentives to both health plans and beneficiaries for efficiency and good decisionmaking. Options that simply increase program revenues or focus only on improving trust fund solvency may seem attractive, but they do not address the fundamental problems facing Medicare.

The popular assumption that the Balanced Budget Act has taken major steps to slow the growth of Medicare spending, coupled with budget surpluses and a booming economy, has sapped political enthusiasm for restructuring the program. Nonetheless, the baby boomers are inexorably approaching the time when they too will expect Medicare coverage. No single policy reform can guarantee that those expectations will be met. Instead, many policy initiatives will be needed over an extended period to adapt the program to the challenges of the new century.

## Notes

1. Based on CBO estimates (1998b, 49). The GDP share of Medicare spending in 1998 is somewhat smaller than the corresponding figure for 1995 reported in that volume.

2. That estimate is based on the intermediate assumptions of the Medicare trustees, as reported by the Board of Trustees of the Federal Hospital Insurance Trust Fund (1999, 13).

3. Excess profits could be returned in the form of a rebate to the federal government, but all plans prefer to offer additional benefits because of the obvious marketing incentive.

## References

Board of Trustees of the Federal Hospital Insurance Trust Fund. 1999. *1999 Annual Report of the Board of Trustees of the Federal Hospital Insurance Trust Fund.* Washington, D.C.: Government Printing Office.

Christensen, Sandra, and Judy Shinogle. 1997. "Effects of Supplemental Coverage on Use of Services by Medicare Enrollees." *Health Care Financing Review*, fall: 5–17.

Congressional Budget Office. 1998a. *An Analysis of the President's Budgetary Proposals for Fiscal Year 1999*. Washington, D.C.: CBO.

———. 1998b. *Long-Term Budgetary Pressures and Policy Options*. Washington, D.C.: CBO.

Cromwell, Jerry, Debra Dayhoff, and Armen Thoumaian. 1997. "Cost Savings and Physician Responses to Global Bundled Payments for Medicare Heart Bypass Surgery." *Health Care Financing Review*, fall: 41–57.

Eppig, Franklin J., and George S. Chulis. 1997. "Trends in Medicare Supplementary Insurance: 1992–1996." *Health Care Financing Review*, fall: 201–6.

Medicare Payment Advisory Commission. 1999. *Report to the Congress: Medicare Payment Policy*. Washington, D.C.: MedPAC.

National Academy of Social Insurance. 1998. *Structuring Medicare Choices*. Washington, D.C.: NASI.

Riley, Gerald, Cynthia Tudor, Yen-Pin Chiang, and Melvin Ingber. 1996. "Health Status of Medicare Enrollees in HMOs and Fee-for-Service in 1994." *Health Care Financing Review*, summer: 65–76.

# 3

# Converting Medicare to Prepaid Health Insurance

Andrew J. Rettenmaier and Thomas R. Saving

In reviewing the national health insurance movement that ultimately led to President Lyndon B. Johnson's signing of the Medicare Act on July 30, 1965, we were struck by the deep understanding of the issues by Wilbur Mills, chairman of the House Committee on Ways and Means at the time. In the years leading up to Medicare's passage, he had resisted any bill that relied on financing through the Social Security system because of his concerns about the actuarial soundness of the proposed Medicare financing arrangements:

> The central fact which must be faced on a proposal to provide a form of service benefit B as contrasted to a cash benefit B is that it is very difficult to accurately estimate the

The authors wish to thank the Lynde and Harry Bradley Foundation and the National Center for Policy Analysis for financial support. They also wish to thank Hugh Richardson and Liqun Liu for their valuable comments and suggestions.

cost. These difficult-to-predict future costs, when such a program is part of the Social Security program, could well have highly dangerous ramifications on the cash benefits portion of the Social Security system.

Further:

In practical terms, this meant that if the hospital insurance system which would be created by the bill was to remain sound, the taxable wage base would have to be increased at least $150 each year. Clearly, this would be a case of the tail wagging the dog. The Congress would be left completely hamstrung, with only two alternatives: (1) A total program which we know was actuarially unsound, or (2) a commitment into the indefinite future to a steady but wholly uncontrolled increase, due to the hospital part of the program, in the amount of wages taxed for social security purposes. Clearly, we could not conscientiously be a party to such an abrogation of congressional responsibility.

He went on to indicate that average earnings in covered employment were growing at a 4 percent annual rate from 1955 to 1963, while average daily hospitalization costs were growing at 6.7 percent annually, and that he had no reason to assume that the growth in hospitalization cost would slow. Mills foresaw that such a system would be actuarially unsound and would generate an unfunded liability by providing hospitalization benefits immediately to individuals who had not paid into the system. Mills articulated this concern and introduced the notion of prepayment or prefunding:

However, on the question of financing, a further very serious problem is the effect which the assumption of the liability for the hospital costs for all of the currently retired persons will have on the Social Security program as a whole. I do not believe that it is generally understood that this unfunded liability would amount to at least $33 billion. It must be realized that the currently retired individuals under the Social Security program have not paid any taxes as such for hospital insurance benefits. This is where the prepayment argument when applied to the King-Anderson proposal completely breaks down. (Mills 1964)

From the outset, it was common knowledge within the Social Security Administration and in Congress that Medicare would face financing difficulties. Nonetheless, by July 1965, an even broader program than the one serving as a point of reference for these comments would become law. Mills would eventually relent and support the passage of the existing Medicare system.[1]

As the past thirty years have shown, Mills's predictions have been on the mark. Between 1967 and 1997, the growth rate in total real Medicare expenditures was 8.12 percent, compared with a 2.22 percent combined real growth rate in wages and workers. The Medicare tax rate and taxable wage base have had to be increased significantly from an initial rate of 0.7 percent and base of $6,600. The payroll tax has been increased numerous times in reaching its current level of 2.9 percent in 1986. The level of earnings subject to the tax rose from $6,600 in 1966 to $135,000 in 1993 and to the current unlimited level in 1994. Despite numerous increases in the effective tax rate, Medicare now pays out more in benefits than it receives in tax revenues.

Medicare and Social Security share a common heritage and structure. They both provide social insurance benefiting the aged population and rely primarily on pay-as-you-go financing. The combination of increased benefits and a generational shock in the form of the baby boomers puts us on the verge of losing a valuable program. The surge in the number of Medicare recipients and the increase in the years each will receive benefits place the system used to finance Medicare under extreme duress. However, the system can be rescued by moving to prepayment. Replacing the generational transfer system of finance with prepayment before the baby boomers retire will provide the resources to cover the retirement expenditures not only of the baby boom generation, but of all generations that follow, regardless of their size.

## Some Theoretical Considerations

It appeared clear from the outset that the Medicare program as enacted would quickly be fully financed by generational transfers. It has long been argued, beginning with Samuelson (1958), that in a growing economy such transfers are welfare-enhancing. Using the construct of an overlapping generations model, such a transfer system is welfare-enhancing because it allows the aging generation to receive a subsidy from either an ever-growing younger population base or an ever-growing technology. The current research on the reform of both Social Security's and Medicare's generational transfer basis argues that the transfer mechanism contains incentive effects that more than offset any welfare gain from the generational transfer. Indeed, opponents of the current system argue that one way to obtain the real resources necessary to pay for the coming retirement of the baby boomers is to remove the disincentive to save. The increase in the level of saving and the resulting increase in the nation's real capital stock would increase the nation's income and help pay for the predicted deficits in both the Social Security and Medicare programs.

Replacing a generational transfer system with a prepaid system must mean that the generational transfer system is inherently inefficient. There is theoretical evidence that a system of lump-sum generational transfers is inferior to a prepaid system. This theoretical inferiority of generational transfer results in both a welfare loss and a decrease in the nation's capital stock. Thus, the movement to a prepaid system of finance could help us over the baby-boom retirement disaster by giving a once-and-for-all bump in output as we move to the larger capital stock inherent in the prepaid equilibrium.

In the appendix, we use a two-period overlapping-generations model to demonstrate that generational transfers are inefficient and that moving to a prepaid system will increase the nation's capital stock and income. We consider consumers with identical preferences and production functions and require that they can transfer consumption from the working period of their lives to their retirements only through the accumulation of capital, that is, by saving. This capital accumulation determines the economy's total output, net of capital depreciation, in any period. The theoretical issue is how this method of distribution of total output, net of depreciation, between the working and retired populations affects the equilibrium of the capital stock and the consumption of the two populations. We compare the solution obtained with prepaid retirement, the laissez-faire solution, with an intergenerational transfer from the working population to the retired population financed by two alternative methods: (1) a lump-sum tax on the working population that is transferred to the retired population and (2) an income tax imposed on the working population that is transferred to the retired population.

In keeping with tradition, we ignore any congestion effects of population size. In the model, we assume that individuals can produce capital at essentially constant costs; this process results in constant returns to economy size, where size refers to the existing capital stock.[2] In equilibrium, for any given population size, the per capita capital stock and consumption are independent of the level of population. Moreover, given the general decline in fertility rates worldwide, generation transfer systems that are based on continual population growth seem doomed to failure. Therefore, we restrict our analysis to a constant population world. The question here is how income and the capital stock in a constant population world are affected by moving from self-financed retirement consumption to retirement consumption financed by generational transfers.

Consider first a generational transfer system financed by a per capita lump-sum tax imposed on the working generation and distributed to the retired generation. Given fairly normal assumptions about preferences and technology, an intergenerational transfer of this kind (from the young to the old) always reduces the equilibrium capital stock.[3] This analysis shows that, even if we achieve the generational transfer with a supposedly nondistortionary lump-sum tax, the per capita capital stock falls, and hence, the level of goods available per capita to both the working and retired generations for consumption is reduced. Moreover, the higher capital price that is associated with the lower capital stock in the generational transfer world further distorts individual choice. Even though the lump-sum tax-financed transfer does not affect the real market opportunities to trade between periods, the higher capital price affects an individual's perceived trade-off between periods.

A relatively simple figure can illustrate the equilibrium lifetime consumption choice to demonstrate that even financing a generational transfer by a lump-sum tax reduces the economy's capital stock. Because only the working generation produces any income, greater desired consumption in an individual's retirement requires a larger capital stock. Up to a point, this increase in the capital allows an individual's consumption during employment and retirement to rise. Eventually, increased consumption during retirement reduces consumption during employment. In figure 3–1, we refer to the trade-off between consumption during employment and consumption during retirement as *trade frontiers*.

This figure depicts the trade frontiers for the prepaid-retirement laissez-faire world and the generational transfer world. The curves labeled *PP*, *TT*, and *T'T'* represent, respectively, the frontier for the prepaid-retirement laissez-faire world (at the original price of capital), the generation transfer world before any change in the price of capital, and the price of a capital-adjusted world (at a new, higher price of capital required to achieve equilibrium in the generational transfer world). Each point on the *TT* curve is derived from a point on the *PP* curve by

## FIGURE 3–1
### EQUILIBRIUM LIFETIME CONSUMPTION

Retired period consumption

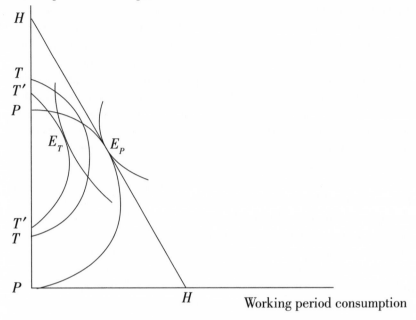

Working period consumption

SOURCE: Rettenmaier and Saving 1999.

subtracting a fixed lump-sum transfer from the working period and adding the same lump-sum transfer to consumption during retirement. Further, because, after a forced transfer of consumption from their employment to their retirement, consumers have too much retirement consumption, the price of capital increases, and the relevant trade frontier shifts to $T'T'$, which is everywhere inside or on the $TT$ curve.

The point $E_p$ in the figure represents the pretransfer steady-state equilibrium levels of consumption in the two periods and either lies to the right of the tangent point of $PP$ or is at that tangent point. The straight line through the point $E_T$ tangent to $PP$ is denoted as $HH$. Thus, $HH$ is strictly to the right of $TT$ and, therefore, to the right of $T'T'$. The point $E_p$ represents the tangent point of the indifference curves and frontier $T'T'$ and identifies the steady-state equilibrium levels of retirement and employment consumption in the transfer world. Because $E_p$ lies strictly outside both frontiers $TT$ and $T'T'$, it strictly dominates point $E_T$. Therefore, moving from the free market world to the transfer world results in a reduction in the capital stock and a permanent reduction in the national income.

Consider a tax more like the payroll tax used to finance both Social Security and Medicare. The most important point is that an intergenerational transfer, regardless of its financing method, always reduces the capital stock. We can rigorously prove that the equilibrium capital price in the income-tax generational transfer world exceeds the price of capital in the prepaid-retirement world. Based on this, we can go on to show that the equilibrium stock of capital in the income-tax generation transfer world is smaller than the stock of capital in the prepaid-retirement world.

Regardless of the financing, individuals are worse off in a world with young-to-old intergenerational transfers than in a laissez-faire world of prepaid retirement. Within the transfer world, the form of financing makes a difference because different financing methods have different economic effects. Intuitively, income tax financing will make intergenerational transfers even less attractive than the lump-sum tax financing because of the identified negative incentive effects of income taxes. But this intuition in favor of the lump-sum tax is no longer correct in an overlapping generations economy.

The results obtained above were based on a behavior model in which the labor supply of the working generation was assumed to be unresponsive to the existence of an intergenerational transfer. Given the level of labor supplied in the prepaid world, we can show that, for that level of labor, the capital stock in the generation transfer world, no matter how financed, is less than in the prepaid-retirement world. In addition, the reduction in the capital stock induced by generation transfer reduces the marginal product of labor and therefore reduces labor supplied. As a result, there is a further reduction in the capital stock, which increases the welfare cost of the transfer. The income tax–financed transfer has the advantage that it treats labor and capital symmetrically and does not have any additional labor market effects.

In general, then, the imposition of a generational transfer system of financing retirement consumption reduces the nation's capital stock and causes a permanent reduction in national income. Thus, reversing this process and moving from the existing generational transfer system used to finance Social Security and Medicare to a prepaid system can be partially paid for through the increase in the capital stock that will accompany the introduction of prepaid-retirement financing.

## A Cohort-Based Solution

Because Medicare is financed by transfer payments from workers to retirees, benefits can grow at the same rate as the tax base, which is a function of wage and population growth, assuming the tax rate is held constant. As Medicare's financing and benefit history has shown, the growth in benefits has far outpaced the growth in real earnings. Congress has had to resort to expanding the tax base and tax rate to keep up with the expenditure growth. Under the status quo, tax rates will have to be increased significantly. As indicated in the previous section, a shift in financing retirement pensions away from transfer payments to prefunding would raise the nation's capital stock and increase individuals' well-being.

Health care is just one type of retirement expense considered in the previous section, but with the institution of Medicare, it has been given separate treatment in the budgets of retirees. Health care in general is afforded preferential treatment in the budgets of a majority of the nonaged population in that health insurance purchased by employers is not taxed. The link between employers and health insurance purchases started during World War II, when increasing labor demand and wage and price controls forced employers to increase worker compensation by means other than wage hikes. At the time, employer-purchased health insurance was not taxed, and that preferential tax status, which changed the relative price of health care, has persisted. Just as important, health care enjoys its elevated status because society has decided that individuals will have access to health care regardless of the ability to pay for it. Nonetheless, the results demonstrated above hold for prefunding health care as well as other expenses during retirement.

Prefunding retirement health care could be accomplished at the cohort level. Each age cohort, defined as all individuals born in a given calendar year, would become a risk pool; a specified contribution would be required of each cohort member. Requiring the participation of all cohort members would address some problems associated with adverse selection and myopic behavior. The contributions accumulated over a lifetime would be used to purchase a basic retirement health insurance policy. Individuals would collect on the insurance if they reached the specified retirement age and if they had health expenditures that exceeded the policy's deductible. In the following simulations, we define the basic policy as one with a $2,500 deductible and full coverage beyond the deductible. We also consider prefunding the basic Medicare policy, net of premium payments. The basic issue is how much health care would be specifically prefunded and how much would be purchased with general retirement-income sources.

Regardless of who ultimately pays for the health care services consumed by the aged, their health care risks will exist. How health care evolves and what proportion of total resources are directed to it are not known. These unknowns do not, however, necessitate that retirement health care be financed with transfer payments. The current financing system shifts the burden of health care risks to the working population, away from the health care consumers. Continuing the system binds generations to a contract that they did not sign. With prefunding, future retirees pay for their own retirement health expenditures rather than relying on future workers.

Prefunding could be executed as follows. Contributions to individual accounts, up to the specified level for the cohort, would reduce payroll tax liability dollar for dollar. Payroll taxes beyond the required contributions would be used to defray part of the transition cost and to pay for the basic insurance of low-income individuals within one's age cohort. Each individual would establish a personal retirement insurance for medical expenses (PRIME) account with an approved provider. Account providers would be subject to reasonable safety requirements. PRIME accounts would differ from medical IRAs in that individuals could draw on the accounts conditional on reaching retirement age. This insurance would be similar to Medicare in that it would pay no death benefit.

Contribution rates would adjust as new information about medical care expenses is revealed. In the aggregate, as each age group reaches retirement age, there would be sufficient funds in the group members' PRIME accounts to cover the insurance premiums of each member. But members of the retiring cohort will have varying medical care expenditure risks. If each cohort member chooses among a set of alternative health care packages, how do we ensure that all levels of risk are serviced?

## Choice and Adverse Selection

By requiring all members of a cohort to participate in funding their health insurance, we have partially addressed adverse selection. However, at retirement, individuals have varying risks—some obvious, some not. The issues involved in allowing choice when all beneficiaries have the same budget but different risks are the same issues facing the current system with the expansion of choices resulting from the provisions in the Balanced Budget Act of 1997. Those issues include the stability of the set of insurance packages in the face of adverse selection and the insurers' screening out high risks within a particular group.

In the prefunded system, if individuals choose their insurer when they enter the labor force at age twenty-two, when they presumably know little about medical care needs during retirement, then they will be dispersed across insurers randomly, and the average endowment will cover the expected expenditures. Insurers would also find it difficult to discern who would and who would not pose the risk of high health expenditures during retirement. Though lifetime contracts go a long way toward solving adverse selection and screening, individual preferences change, and the lack of choice at retirement may not provide sufficient freedom.

Shorter contract periods can help solve the asymmetric information and screening problems. Insurance coverage could be chosen at retirement and fixed for the rest of the individual's life. A policy that runs the length of retirement may reduce adverse-selection problems in several ways. First, there is less information. Specifically, there is less known at age 65 about the timing and the magnitude of health care expenditures over the rest of a beneficiary's life than is known about possible expenditures next year. Second, the important cost is the expected present value of the individual's remaining lifetime health expenses. It is no longer obvious how these vary with health, as sicker people generally die earlier and spend less on health care. Insurers would be confronted with both health care risk and longevity risk. Figure 3–2 gives the present value of annual Medicare payments for individuals who die at ages 65 to 100, with three discount rates: 3 percent, 5 percent, and 7 percent. In present value terms, individuals who die at young ages and old ages have comparable present values of their payments. Therefore, screening on the part of insurers would be much more difficult if the insurance contract is initiated at age 65 and runs over the entirety of an enrollee's life.

Long-term contracts would also work to reduce the "inequality" in the claims distribution compared with the dispersion of claims over shorter periods. Thus, even with choice at the initiation of the contracts, insurers would face similar distributions of expected claims. On reaching retirement, all individuals in a cohort would sign up for health insurance and would place their entire account in the hands of a health insurer. With this feature, consumer choice after the contracts were ini-

## FIGURE 3–2

PRESENT VALUE OF MEDICARE PAYMENT AT AGE SIXTY-FIVE, BY AGE AT DEATH

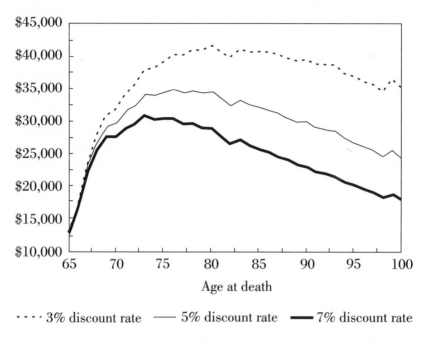

Age at death

- - - - 3% discount rate   ——— 5% discount rate   ━━━ 7% discount rate

SOURCE: The annual benefit profiles on which the present values in the figure are based come from the data used in producing the graphs in Lubitz, Beebe, and Baker 1995.

tiated would be possible. As Cochrane (1995) shows, contracts that included severance payments would solve both the renewability and the adverse-selection problem. If an individual's health status fell, and thus was likely to incur higher costs of care, the insurer would have to make a payment to the individual equal to the expected increase in benefits to be paid, in the event that the individual wanted to switch insurers. The expected value of the individuals' benefit payments, based on new information, is equal to the amount another insurer would require to enter its pool. The new present value is also the amount the current insurer expects to spend on the individual and is therefore willing to spend to be released from the obligation. Because the amount is the same, individuals are free to move between insurers. If, conversely, an individual experienced a positive health shock and desired to switch insurers, the individual would take along the reduced present value of future health care benefits. In this way, nonhealth-related consumption would be unaffected by shocks to health status.

## The Cost of Prefunded Insurance

The next step in discussing a prefunded system of retirement medical insurance is to identify the cost of insurance. We calculate the contribution rates that would be necessary for each age cohort to prefund its retirement medical care. The equation below identifies the contribution rate as the ratio of the present value of expected future benefits to the present value of expected life-cycle earnings,

$$
C_{a_0} = \frac{\displaystyle\sum_{t = 65 - a_0}^{119 - a_0} \frac{p_{a_0,t} \, b_{a_0,t}}{(1 + r)^t}}{\displaystyle\sum_{t = 0}^{64 - a_0} \frac{p_{a_0,t} \, y_{a_0,t}}{(1 + r)^t}} \tag{3-1}
$$

where $a_0$ is the cohort's age at the beginning of a transition to a prefunded program, $C_{a_0}$ is the percentage of remaining lifetime earnings that must be saved to purchase retirement medical insurance given age $a_0$, $y_{a_0,t}$ is the mean real income for cohort $a_0$ in year $t$, $r$ is the real interest rate, $b_{a_0,t}$ is the mean real retirement medical care insurance premium for cohort $a_0$ in year $t$, and $p_{a_0,t}$ is the probability of surviving to year $t$ for an individual of age $a_0$. Given this interpretation, $p_{a_0,t} = \Pi_{i + a_0}^{a_0 + t} s_i$, where $s_i$ is the probability of surviving from $\text{age}_i$ to $\text{age}_{i+1}$.

The projected life-cycle earnings by birth cohort, which serve as the denominator in the estimates of the contribution rate, are based on historical growth rates of the three components of annual earnings: participation, hours, and hourly wage. We estimated growth rates by sex, age, and education categories by using historical data from the 1964 to 1996 March supplements to the Current Population Surveys. For a detailed description of how each earnings component was forecasted and a comparison among alternatives, see Rettenmaier and Saving 1999. The mortality rates are the Census Bureau's middle series. The 1995, 2005, and 2050 life tables are used along with linear interpolations by age for the intervening years and for years beyond 2050 to produce cohort-specific life tables.

TABLE 3–1

REQUIRED CONTRIBUTION RATES EXPRESSED AS A PERCENTAGE OF
LIFE-CYCLE EARNINGS

| *Real Rate of Return* | *Medical Expenditures Growth* | *Medicare Benefits Net of Premiums* | *$2,500 Deductible Policy* |
|---|---|---|---|
| 3.5 | 1 | 4.37 | 3.69 |
| 3.5 | 2 | 7.65 | 6.44 |
| 5.4 | 1 | 2.19 | 1.85 |
| 5.4 | 2 | 3.77 | 3.19 |
| 6.4 | 1 | 1.52 | 1.29 |
| 6.4 | 2 | 2.61 | 2.21 |
| 9.0 | 1 | 0.59 | 0.51 |
| 9.0 | 2 | 1.00 | 0.85 |

SOURCE: Authors' calculations.

The benefits series for ages sixty-five and beyond, which form the numerator in the calculation of the contribution rate, are based on data from the Health Care Financing Administration's (HCFA) 1995 Cost and Use File. The Cost and Use File combines information from the Medicare Current Beneficiary Survey and HCFA's administration files to produce detailed expenditure records. Contribution rates for two benefit series are reported in table 3–1. For the first set of estimates, $b_{a_0,t}$ is based on the weighted average of Part A and Part B benefits net of premium payments by age. The second set of estimates is based on the price of the $2,500 deductible policy. The price is estimated by applying the RAND Health Insurance Experiment simulation results, reported in Keeler and colleagues 1988, to the total expenditures of each individual in an age group. Because Medicare's two-part structure does not fit precisely into the simulation result, we estimate several effects of the higher deductible on total expenditures, depending on the type of supplemental insurance. A description of how the RAND simulation results were applied to the expenditure data can also be found in Rettenmaier and Saving 1999.

The historical rate of return on capital has exceeded the rate of growth that can be expected from a pay-as-you-go system with the current fertility rates. Poterba and Samwick (1995) calculated a real pretax rate of return on capital in the nonfinancial corporate sector of 9.2 percent for the years 1947 through 1995. Feldstein and Samwick (1997) estimate that a portfolio "of 60 percent equity and 40 percent debt had a yield of about 5.5 percent over both the postwar period and the period since 1926." They also suggest that if corporate taxes at all levels take 40 percent of pretax debt and equity income, then a 5.4 percent after-tax return is equivalent to a 9 percent pretax return. Based on the Standard & Poor's 500, including dividend reinvestment, from 1926 to 1995, a 100 percent equity portfolio would have earned a real rate of return equal to 6.4 percent. We account for all these estimates by estimating the two levels of the contribution rate required to prefund retirement health care with a conservative 3.5 percent real rate of return, the after-tax 5.4 percent rate and the pretax 9 percent rate on a portfolio of equities and bonds, and the after-tax rate of 6.4 percent on an equity portfolio.

Two real growth rates in per capita medical care expenditures, 1 and 2 percent, are considered. By way of comparison, the Medicare trustees in 1998 assumed that Medicare's real cost per unit of service would grow at a rate of about 1 percent during the five years of the forecast, would rise to 3.5 percent for the next eight years, and then would gradually decline to approximately 0.9 percent by the twenty-fifth year and continue at that rate over the remaining years of the projection. The trustees' assumptions fall in between the two shown in table 3–1.

Table 3–1 presents the lifetime contribution rates that the average new entrants to the labor force would face under the various assumptions about the rate of return on their investments, the growth rate in medical care expenditures, and the cost of the benefits being prefunded. The contribution rate for entering cohorts ranges from a low of 0.51 percent to a high of 7.65 percent, depending on the cost and growth rate assumptions. In 1998, Medicare's total expenditures, net of premium payments, associated with treating the population sixty-five and older represented an amount that would equal 4.24 percent of taxable payroll. The contribution rates are less than the implied tax rate for all but the most pessimistic set of assumptions in table 3–1. Thus, if the 4.24 percent tax were maintained, new entrants could fund their retirement medical care and have some tax left over to fund the cost of the transition.

## Comparing the Current System to a Prefunded System

The stumbling block to prefunding, however, is the transition cost. A transition involves the same set of issues with which Wilbur Mills and other members of Congress wrestled before Medicare's passage and which were faced by the Congresses between 1937 and 1950, in Social Security's early years. In both instances, transfer-payment financing was chosen instead of waiting to prefund the system or imposing higher taxes during the startup phase. During the transition to a prefunded system, the commitments to the currently retired population and those close to the retirement age must be funded, and the contributions to cohort accounts must be made.

However, younger workers can prefund their retirement insurance at rates less than the current implied tax rate. Thus, part of the transition cost would be offset by the difference between the implied tax rate and the cohort contribution rate. In the example below, we assume a real rate of return of 5.4 percent and real per capita medical expenditures growth of 1 percent. Present values of the status quo and transition liabilities are calculated with the 2.8 percent rate of return on government bonds in the 1998 trustees' report.

A transition could be structured in the following way. The current implied tax rate remains in effect out to the last year in the simulation, 2080. We evaluate the case in which all baby boomers are shifted to the new system; thus, everyone born in 1946 and later is in the new system, while individuals older than fifty-two in 1998 remain in the old system. With this structure, the expenses associated with the transition are the same as the expenses associated with maintaining the current system out to the year 2010. Beyond 2010, no new beneficiaries are added to the old system. The only beneficiaries in the old system are those cohorts born in 1945 and earlier, which results in continuously declining expenses beyond 2010.

Table 3–2 gives the present values of a transition and of maintaining the current system and shows the oldest cohort that could prefund retirement health insurance with a contribution rate less than 4.24 percent. As seen in the first row, new entrants to the labor force can prefund retirement medical expenses for 1.85 percent of their lifetime earnings. This option leaves 2.39 percent (4.24 − 1.85) of their earnings available to defray the transition cost associated with paying the Medicare costs of those who remain in the system. Since individuals younger than forty-two can fund their own retirement medical insurance for less than 4.24 percent of their remaining lifetime earnings, they all are contributing toward the retirement health insurance of those in the old system and those older than forty-two in the new system. Contributions to the cohort-based insurance that are for individuals between forty-three and fifty-two and that are

TABLE 3–2

TRANSITION COST ESTIMATES IN BILLIONS ASSUMING 5.4 PERCENT
REAL RATE OF RETURN AND 1 PERCENT REAL GROWTH IN
PER CAPITA MEDICAL EXPENDITURES

| | | | Present Value of Unfunded Liability | |
| | Tax Rate | Switch | | |
| Benefit Estimate | at 22 | Age[a] | Status quo | Transition |
|---|---|---|---|---|
| $2,500 deductible policy | 1.85 | 42 | $5,566 | $841 |
| Medicare benefits net of premiums | 2.19 | 39 | $5,566 | $1,640 |

a. The switch age designates the oldest cohort able to fund retirement medical care for <4.24% of lifetime earnings.
SOURCE: Authors' calculations.

in excess of the 4.24 percent implied tax are counted against the transition tax revenues, but all tax revenues collected from the population fifty-three and older would be counted as transition tax revenues.

The first row in table 3–2 indicates that a transition to a funded system of high-deductible insurance policies can be accomplished for about 15 percent of the cost of maintaining the status quo. The present value of the unfunded liability for the status quo is $5.6 trillion under these assumptions, and the present value of the transition liability is $841 billion. Replacing Medicare benefits, net of Part B premiums, could be accomplished for less than 30 percent of maintaining the status quo, as indicated in the bottom row in table 3–2. The additional cost of the two transition scenarios could be covered by tax increases of 0.46 and 0.90 percent, respectively, which would remain in effect out to the year 2080. These tax increases compare with a tax increase of 3.60 percent, which would be necessary to maintain the status quo under the same assumptions.

These results illustrate the relative costs of the prefunded and the pay-as-you-go systems. Figure 3–3 presents the revenues and expenditures for the case in which Medicare, net of premium payments, is prefunded by the individuals in the new system. In this example, the transition runs a deficit for the first thirty years, but beginning in 2028 and continuing for all future periods, the transition runs a surplus. Under the same set of assumptions, pay-as-you-go revenues would cover

FIGURE 3–3

SYSTEM COSTS AND TAX REVENUES, 1998–2050

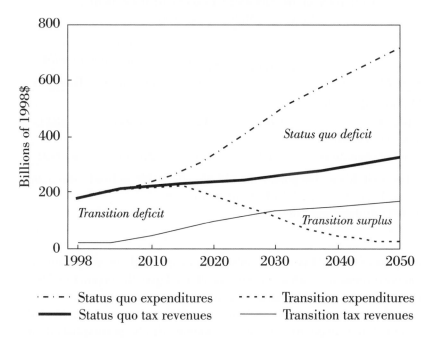

SOURCE: Authors' calculations.

expenditures for the first few years and would fall short of expenditures in all remaining periods.

The primary point of this example is to illustrate the relative costs of prefunding and pay-as-you-go financing. The present values of prefunding exceed those of pay-as-you-go. A transition could be financed with additional government borrowing in the initial periods. Such borrowing would be implemented through a sinking fund with debenture bonds. Payments on the bonds could be made as the transition revenues begin to exceed expenditures. An alternative would be to require individuals to contribute to PRIME accounts in addition to paying the implied taxes. This option would release future generations from tax liabilities, but current workers would pay more. An intermediate approach, which we have taken, is to raise taxes immediately by the amount necessary to make the prefunded system solvent. Because the implied tax rate of 4.70–5.14 percent is maintained indefinitely, the transition is fairly neutral in its effects across generations. These rates are below those necessary to maintain the status quo in the near future. Over time, the capital stock would gradually rise and would increase the nation's income.

## Conclusion

Solving the Medicare crisis is in many ways related to solving the Social Security crisis, but Medicare also has unique features that require unique solutions. Most Medicare reforms are aimed at reducing the cost of providing care to the current beneficiaries and at reducing the rate of growth in per capita expenditures. The system's funding arrangement is often ignored in the reform discussion. But prefunding retirement medical insurance deserves serious consideration, particularly at this time, when prefunding retirement pensions is being debated.

The attempt to correct an earlier form of financing mistake is compounded by the baby boom generation. The retirement of the baby boomers, beginning in 2011, will give the elderly a much greater weight in the population distribution. As a result, the elderly will be consuming a greater share of the gross domestic product than at any previous time in our history. The question is not whether the elderly's share of all consumption will rise—it will. But how will we compel the younger generations to consume less so that the elderly can consume more? We can hope for a windfall in the form of a technological change that will suddenly increase gross domestic product and solve our problem. Or, more realistically, we can do something now that will increase the size of the pie and therefore reduce the pain inflicted on younger generations by the increased consumption of the elderly. Moving from generational transfer financing to prepayment financing will increase the capital stock and therefore increase future GDP. We can make our own windfall.

Prefunding also establishes individuals' ownership of their retirement medical insurance in a way that cannot be accomplished with transfer-payment financing. This notion runs counter to the arguments made by Wilbur Cohen, one of the most ardent early supporters of a payroll tax to finance Medicare, when he stated: "This gives beneficiaries the psychological feeling that they have helped to pay for their protection. It is the reason why Social Security has been so popular and well accepted. People do not want something that is called a hand-out or welfare" (Brownlee 1996, 149). Rather than giving beneficiaries the psychological feeling that they have helped pay for their protection, pre-funding with individual ownership establishes that beneficiaries *have* paid for their protection and that it belongs to them.

## Appendix

Consider a simple, two-period overlapping-generations model in which all consumers have identical preferences. For a consumer born in period $t$, the model is written as

$$U = U(c_t^t, c_t^{t+1}). \tag{3A-1}$$

Let each consumer have one unit of labor to supply in the first period of life and then retire in the second period. Assume further that only capital can be carried over from period to period. Therefore, consumers accumulate capital in the first period and use that capital to purchase consumption during the last period of their life.

On the production side, assume that each individual has a production function that, given the one unit of labor available in period $t$ and using capital purchased from the retired generation, permits the production of output that can be designated on a once-and-for-all basis as either capital or consumption. Denote this production function as

$$y_t = f(k_t) \tag{3A-2}$$

where $y_t$, $k_t$ are, respectively, output and the capital stock purchased by the representative consumer in period $t$.[4] Thus, at any time, individuals can add to their stock of purchased capital by consuming less so that behavior is constrained by

$$y_t = c_t^t + P_t k_t + \Delta k_t = f(k_t) \tag{3A-3}$$

where $P_t$ is the period $t$ price of capital in terms of consumption units and $\Delta k_t$ is the contemporaneous production of capital. Assuming a constant rate of capital depreciation, $\delta$, consumption in period $t + 1$ for generation $t$ individuals is

$$c_t^{t+1} = P_{t+1}[k_t + (\Delta k_t - \delta k_t)]. \tag{3A-4}$$

To maximize lifetime utility, the representative consumer of generation $t$ decides at the beginning of time $t$ how much productive capital to purchase $(k_t)$ and how much additional capital to produce $(\Delta k_t)$, which then determines consumption at $t + 1$, given the capital prices in both periods. In choosing $k_t$ and $\Delta k_t$, current and future consumption $c_t^t$ and $c_t^{t+1}$ are simultaneously determined through the budget constraints, equations 3A–3 and 3A–4.

Given that the economy is in the steady state, the following three equations characterize the equilibrium:

$$c_t^t + c_t^{t+1} = f\left(\frac{c_t^{t+1}}{P}\right) - \delta \, \frac{c_t^{t+1}}{P}$$

$$\frac{U_{c_t^{t+1}}}{U_{c_t^t}} = \frac{1}{P}$$

(3A–5)

$$P = f'\left(\frac{c_t^{t+1}}{P}\right) + 1 - \delta.$$

Equations 3A–5 fully characterize the steady-state competitive equilibrium level of $c_t^t$, $c_t^{t+1}$, and $P$ with the equilibrium per capita capital stock being $k_t = c_t^{t+1}/P$.[5] We now discuss two methods of intergenerational transfers: lump-sum–financed transfers and income-tax–financed transfers. The equilibrium per capita capital stock for each of these forms of financing an intergenerational transfer will be compared with the competitive equilibrium per capita capital stock.

## Lump-Sum–Financed Transfers

Because the basic model has no congestion effects, there are constant returns to economy size. Thus, when the population is constant and the last periods' consumption is prefinanced through capital purchases in the prior period, the per capita capital stock and consumption are independent of the level of population. Moreover, prefunded retirement consumption benefits from population growth through the equilibrium price of capital.[6]

Assume that a generational transfer system is introduced, financed with a per capita lump-sum tax, $T$, imposed on generation $t$, the working generation, and distributed to generation $t - 1$, the retired generation.

This lump-sum-tax–financed intergenerational transfer requires changing budget constraints, equations 3A–3 and 3A–4, respectively, to

$$c_t^t + P_t k_t + \Delta k_t = f(k_t) - T \tag{3A-3'}$$

$$c_t^{t+1} = P_{t+1}[k_t + (\Delta k_t - \delta k_t)] + T. \tag{3A-4'}$$

Accordingly, the steady-state–equilibrium–characterizing conditions become

$$c_t^t + c_t^{t+1} = f\left(\frac{c_t^{t+1} - T}{P_T}\right) - \delta\left(\frac{c_t^{t+1} - T}{P_T}\right)$$

$$\frac{U_{c_t^{t+1}}}{U_{c_t^t}} = \frac{1}{P_T}$$

$$P_T = f'\left(\frac{c_t^{t+1} - T}{P_T}\right) + 1 - \delta \tag{3A-6}$$

where $P_T$ denotes the equilibrium price of capital under a lump-sum tax-financed transfer.

The economic effects and welfare implication of a lump-sum intergenerational transfer amount to a comparison of equations 3A–6 with 3A–5. By comparing the last equation of 3A–5 and the last equation of 3A–6, it is easily shown that, under fairly normal assumptions on preferences and technology, an intergenerational transfer of this kind (from young to the old) always reduces the equilibrium capital stock, hence, $P_T > P$.[7]

The striking result of this analysis is that even if we achieve the generational transfer with a supposedly nondistortionary tax, the result is a reduction in the per capita capital stock and hence reduced per capita goods available for consumption to both generations at time $t$, $(c_t^t + c_t^{t+1})$. Moreover, the higher capital price associated with the lower capital stock in the transfer world further distorts individuals' choice. Even though the lump-sum tax-financed transfer does not affect the real market opportunities to trade between period $t$ consumption and period $t + 1$ consumption, which is one for one, the higher capital price affects an individual's perceived trade-off between period $t$ and period $t + 1$ consumption, which is one for $P$.

## Income-Tax–Financed Transfers

When an intergenerational transfer of size $T$ per person is financed through a proportional income tax, $\tau$, the (steady-state) equilibrium-characterizing conditions become

$$c_t^t + c_t^{t+1} = f\left(\frac{c_t^{t+1} - T}{P_\tau}\right) - \delta\left(\frac{c_t^{t+1} - T}{P_\tau}\right)$$

$$\frac{U_{c_t^{t+1}}}{U_{c_t^t}} = \frac{1}{P_\tau}$$

$$P_\tau = 1 + (1 - \tau)\left[f'\left(\frac{c_t^{t+1} - T}{P_\tau}\right) - \delta\right] \qquad (3A–7)$$

$$\tau\left[f\left(\frac{c_t^{t+1} - T}{P_\tau}\right) - \delta\left(\frac{c_t^{t+1} - T}{P_\tau}\right)\right] = T$$

where $P_\tau$ is the steady-state equilibrium price of capital when the intergenerational transfer is financed by income tax.

The relative performance of the income-tax–financed intergenerational transfer as compared with the laissez-faire and lump-sum tax-financed transfer is, of course, determined by the solution to equations 3A–7 as compared with 3A–5 and 3A–6, respectively. Most important, an intergenerational transfer, regardless of its financing method, is always welfare reducing. It can be rigorously proved that $P_\tau$, the equilibrium price in the income-tax world, is greater than the equilibrium capital price in the laissez-faire world. Based on this, we can give a similar graphical presentation demonstrating that an intergenerational transfer financed by an income tax is also welfare reducing.

We have now established that no matter what kind of financing is used, individuals are worse off in a world with young-to-old intergenerational transfers than in the laissez-faire world. Obviously, within the transfer world, the form of financing makes a difference because different financing methods have different economic effects. Intuitively, income-tax financing will make intergenerational transfers even less attractive than the lump-sum tax financing because of the identified negative incentive effects of income taxes. However, this intuition in favor of the lump-sum tax is no longer correct in an overlapping generations economy.

**Intergenerational Transfers with Variable Labor Supply.** The behavior model used above assumed that utility was not a function of labor supplied in either period. To account for the incentive effects of taxation on labor supplied, we assume that utility is also affected by the level of leisure in the first period (we maintain the assumption that the individual is fully retired in the second period).[8] Denote the level of leisure demanded by a $t$-generation individual in period $t$ as $l_t$ and let the utility function for each individual be

$$U = U(c_t^t, c_t^{t+1}, l_t). \tag{3A-8}$$

The per capita output at time $t$ is

$$(1 - l_t) f\left(\frac{k_t}{1 - l_t}\right) \tag{3A-9}$$

where $k_t$ is still per capita capital stock.[9]

In a world without any transfer, the budget constraints facing a representative generation $t$ individual are

$$c_t^t + P_t k_t + \Delta k_t = (1 - l_t) f\left(\frac{k_t}{1 - l_t}\right)$$

$$c_t^{t+1} = P_{t+1}\left[k_t + (\Delta k_t - \delta k_t)\right]. \tag{3A-10}$$

Proceeding to the steady state, the following equations characterize the equilibrium values of the relevant variables,

$$c_t^t + c_t^{t+1} = (1 - l) f\left(\frac{k}{1 - l}\right) - \delta k$$

$$\frac{U_{c_t^{t+1}}}{U_{c_t^t}} = \frac{1}{P}$$

$$\frac{U_{l_t}}{U_{c_t^t}} = f\left(\frac{k}{1 - l}\right) - \left(\frac{k}{1 - l}\right) f'\left(\frac{k}{1 - l}\right)$$

$$P = f'\left(\frac{k}{1 - l}\right) + (1 - \delta)$$

$$c_t^{t+1} = Pk. \tag{3A-11}$$

Without loss of generality, we can simply define the labor supplied in equilibrium as unity. Thus, the equilibrium conditions for this problem are identical to those for the problem considered above once the optimal labor supply is determined. We shall use this characteristic of the equilibrium in the discussion below.

The two critical equations characterizing the steady state with an intergenerational transfer of size $T$ that is financed by lump-sum tax and by an income tax are, respectively,

$$\frac{U_l}{U_{c_t^t}} = f\left(\frac{c_t^{t+1}-T}{P_T(1-l)}\right) - \left(\frac{c_t^{t+1}-T}{P_T(1-l)}\right) f'\left(\frac{c_t^{t+1}-T}{P_T(1-l)}\right)$$

$$P_T = 1 + \left[f'\left(\frac{c_t^{t+1}-T}{P_T(1-l)}\right) - \delta\right]$$

(3A–12)

$$\frac{U_l}{U_{c_t^t}} = (1-\tau)\left[f\left(\frac{c_t^{t+1}-T}{P_\tau(1-l)}\right) - \left(\frac{c_t^{t+1}-T}{P_\tau(1-l)}\right) f'\left(\frac{c_t^{t+1}-T}{P_\tau(1-l)}\right)\right]$$

$$P_\tau = (1-\tau)\left[f'\left(\frac{c_t^{t+1}-T}{P_\tau(1-l)}\right) - \delta\right] + (1-\delta).$$

Given the level of labor supplied in the prepaid world, $\hat{L}$, we have that $P_{T\hat{L}} > P_{\tau\hat{L}} > P$ and that $k_{T\hat{L}} < k_{\tau\hat{L}} < k$. Consider the first two equations in 3A–12. The transfer-induced reduction in the capital stock reduces the marginal product of labor, the right-hand side of the first equation of 3A–12, and, therefore, reduces labor supplied. As a result, there is a further reduction in the capital stock, which increases the welfare cost of the transfer. Interestingly, the income-tax–financed transfer has the advantage that it treats labor and capital symmetrically and does not have any additional labor market effects.

## Notes

1. See Derthick 1979, 328–34, for a discussion of how the original bill being backed by the Johnson administration, which primarily covered hospitalization insurance, was expanded to include what is now referred to as supplementary medical insurance and the role Mills played in the final negotiations.

2. Models based on continual population growth assume that there is no bound to the capacity of the earth to support human population. That is equivalent to a bacterial growth model in a petri dish of infinite size.

3. The appendix details the analysis underlying this result.

4. Consistent with the current literature, the production function is assumed to be derived from a linear homogeneous function in capital and labor, which can be written as $y_t = L_t F(k_t, 1) = f(k_t)$ since $L_t \equiv 1$.

5. While the social planner's problem would result in maximizing $c_t^t + c_t^{t+1}$, which requires that $f' = \delta$, there is no guarantee that the competitive solution will attain this result. As we show below, however, any implementation of transfers by a social planner results in a reduction in the per capita capital stock and community welfare.

6. Specifically, with a constant population growth rate of $n$, the equilibrium price of capital is $(1 + n)P_0$, where $P_0$ is the zero population growth price of capital. This higher price of capital allows the prepaid retirement to yield a greater return with population growth.

7. In particular, the assumption of the absence of perverse time preference, defined as a preference for the future when consumption in both periods is equal, is sufficient but not necessary for this result.

8. Because we do not consider second-period labor supply, our analysis will not shed light on the retirement decision. For demonstrating the nonoptimality of intergenerational transfers, discussion of the retirement decision is not required, although this decision is important for the financing of retirement consumption.

9. Production specification 3A–9 captures the dependence of output on labor supplied and capital labor ratio, and it is derived from a linearly homogeneous aggregate production function.

# References

Board of Trustees of the Federal Hospital Insurance Trust Fund. 1998. *1998 Annual Report of the Board of Trustees of the Federal Hospital Insurance Trust Fund*. Washington, D.C.: Government Printing Office.

Board of Trustees of the Federal Old-Age and Survivors Insurance and Disability Insurance Trust Funds. 1998. *1998 Annual Report of the Board of Trustees of the Federal Old-Age and Survivors Insurance and Disability Insurance Trust Funds*. Washington, D.C.: Government Printing Office.

Board of Trustees of the Federal Supplementary Medical Insurance Trust Fund. 1998. *1998 Annual Report of the Board of Trustees of the Federal Supple-*

*mentary Medical Insurance Trust Fund*. Washington, D.C.: Government Printing Office.

Brownlee, W. E. 1996. *Funding the Modern American State, 1941–1995: The Rise and Fall of the Era of Easy Finance*. New York: Cambridge University Press.

Cochrane, John H. 1995. "Time Consistent Health Insurance." *Journal of Political Economy* 103 (3) (June): 445–73.

Derthick, Martha. 1979. *Policy Making for Social Security*. Washington, D.C.: Brookings Institution.

Feldstein, Martin, and Andrew Samwick. 1997. "The Economics of Prefunding Social Security and Medicare Benefits." NBER Working Paper 6055.

Keeler, Emmett B., Joan L. Buchanan, John E. Rolph, Janet M. Hanley, and David M. Reboussin. 1988. "The Demand for Episodes of Medical Treatment in the Health Insurance Experiment." RAND Corporation, March.

Lubitz, James, James Beebe, and Colin Baker. 1995. "Longevity and Medicare Expenditures." *New England Journal of Medicine* 332 (15) (April 13): 999–1003.

Mills, Wilbur. 1964. September 24, 1964, speech to the Arkansas–Missouri District Kiwanis Convention. 88th Cong., *Congressional Record*, September 9–October 3, reel 10, University Microfilms, Ann Arbor, Mich.

Poterba, James M., and Andrew Samwick. 1995. "Stock Ownership Pattern, Stock Market Fluctuations, and Consumption." *Brookings Papers on Economic Activity* 2: 295–357.

Rettenmaier, Andrew J., and Thomas R. Saving. 1999. *The Economics of Medicare Reform*. Kalamazoo, Mich.: W. E. Upjohn Institute for Employment Research.

Samuelson, Paul A. 1958. "An Exact Consumption-Loan Model of Interest with or without Social Contrivance of Money." *Journal of Political Economy* 66: 467–82.

# 4

## Can Beneficiaries
## Save Medicare?

### Mark V. Pauly

M edicare is a social insurance covering a predetermined fraction of the costs of certain medical services and thus limiting
the medical-expense risk of those eligible for coverage.
Medicare's primary goal was encouraging the additional use of medical
services, because a lack of insurance was considered a barrier to those
services for many. But this system cannot be sustained into the twenty-
first century at current tax rates and current beneficiary premiums. If
we rule out increased taxes and quasi-taxes (mandatory contributions) on
workers to cover the costs of care for current retirees, can anything be
done to avoid drastic cutbacks in health care and health insurance spending, relative to projected levels of costs? In this chapter I explore the
possibility that higher-income or wealthy beneficiaries assume more financing of their own medical care. Such steps redistribute some burden
from workers and general taxpayers to the well-off elderly and may also
allow the rest of the Medicare system, which has benefited the majority
of elders, to continue access to decent amounts and types of care.

Over the next twenty years, some things, relative to current projections of Medicare benefits and spending, must be sacrificed if taxes

on the nonelderly are not to rise to highly distorted and politically unpalatable levels. How large the sacrifices and who should bear their effects are ultimately value judgments to be made through the political process. Here I outline alternatives, all of which involve increasing the amount that higher-income Medicare beneficiaries pay toward their own medical care and reduce their government subsidy. A more detailed version of the theory supporting these arguments has appeared elsewhere (Pauly 1998); in this chapter I present the argument in more concrete terms and consider some other issues in Medicare reform.

## Are There Alternatives?

Two alternatives can reduce the burden on the tax-financed Medicare system: (1) the use of forced savings and mandated private-insurance coverage, along with cuts in provider payments, and (2) only cuts in provider payments. Both alternatives, though possibly desirable and potentially consistent with beneficiary cost-sharing, are not in themselves the best way to produce the required changes. These two changes are, respectively, current policy favorites of the Right and of the Left.

**Savings instead of Pay-As-You-Go (PAYGO).** Medicare (as well as Social Security) has used payroll taxes on workers to fund current benefits; Medicare also uses general revenue taxes to finance the lion's share of Part B spending. Senator Phil Gramm, Andrew Rettenmaier, and Thomas Saving (1998) recently proposed replacing the PAYGO system with a set of compulsory payroll-tax–funded savings accounts for nonpoor employees. Contributions to these funds during one's working lifetime, plus interest, would solve the Part A trust fund problem, because such contributions—at rates no higher than current Part A tax rates—could finance a uniform catastrophic insurance policy for elders at retirement. This new insurance plan covers a somewhat smaller share of the cost of care than current Medicare does; the benefits are thereby reduced to a level that the taxes can support. This scheme has two main advantages. Because it allows contributions to remain in an account that earns interest rather than being disbursed immediately, it apparently lowers the burden on current workers more than payroll-tax PAYGO financing does. Because each nonpoor citizen pays for his own postretirement health insurance, this payment is independent of the number of retirees and does not vary as the ratio of workers to retirees changes. The proposal offers relatively few details on how competitive markets would be structured to transform savings funds into insurance and provides little explanation of the amount of the deductible or the extent of compulsory coverage; the financing of whatever coverage is specified takes center stage. Along with the relatively low compulsory insurance benefits, the power of compound interest helps substantially to give the proposed program a low tax cost.

The costs quoted, however, will be incurred after the current liability is covered for current and future beneficiaries who are already old enough to have paid low taxes. (In the estimates provided, that will take fifty years, until 2048.) Indeed, the main difference between this savings and investment scheme and the continuation of PAYGO is the pattern of relative burdens imposed on workers when the new scheme is implemented and subsequent costs. Were the savings and investment scheme to be implemented today, compulsory payments (taxes, by any other name) today would be higher than under PAYGO, but eventually they would be lower. The overall burden (in present value terms) of a benefit for current retirees is the same under either scheme, but the savings and investment approach bites the bullet earlier and has lower taxes later than under the PAYGO "crisis." The political feasibility of high taxes to cover transfers remains an issue: the only choice is whether we confront it today or have our children confront it.

To see why this is true, consider the following simple example. Suppose there are three generations: the older generation about to retire (over the next fifteen years or so), the younger generation who will work (and pay taxes or compulsory payments) over forty or more years, and a third generation, just now being born, who will be working when the younger generation retires.

Under PAYGO the younger generation must pay taxes to fund the Medicare and retirement expenses of the older generation; when the younger generation itself retires, its benefits will come from taxes paid by the third generation. Contrast this with the savings and investment scheme. The younger generation will have two obligations. It must continue to pay taxes to pay off the older generation's Medicare benefits, and it must make compulsory savings payments to support its own Medicare benefits. Because interest will be earned on the latter, its payments in the current period will be less than the obligation for eventual benefits. When the younger generation retires, the third generation will not have to pay for the parents' Medicare but will instead need only the lower contemporaneous payments to fund its own medical care expenses.

Comparing the two schemes, we see that the first generation is as well off under either. The third generation would be better off under the savings and investment plan. However, under savings and investment, the second generation is hit twice: not only does it have to pay for its own Medicare, but it has to pay off the older generation. In contrast, under PAYGO the second generation has only to pay off the older generation; its own medical expenses are covered by its children.

In a macroeconomically relevant (but not, obviously, politically meaningful) sense, the savings and investment strategy is better than PAYGO: PAYGO leads to insufficient savings, because the promise of Medicare (and of Social Security) substitutes for true savings. The new scheme forces those savings to occur. The problem is that the savings and investment scheme must either impose the burden of transition on the younger generation or deprive the older generation of benefits— either result will be politically awkward. (The real political question, one suspects, is how attractive the "solve-it-once-and-for-all-and-don't-burden-your-great-grandchildren" slogan will be when real money has to be paid.)

I propose a way of reducing the size of the payoff needed to be made to the current generation, along with a way of reducing the compulsory, government-determined burden on the younger generation. In this sense, my proposal that Medicare beneficiaries who can pay for more of their benefits do so is highly compatible with and will enhance the feasibility of the savings and investment scheme. At present in that scheme, the description of the insurance to be purchased is underdeveloped and poorly attuned to the real purpose of Medicare—which is to get people to use proper amounts of medical care, not to get them to save. The discussion here fleshes out that portion of a reform plan in accord with the approach of the savings and investment scheme.

**Cutting Provider Payments.** The other approach to reducing Medicare outlays and holding the line on taxes is through reducing provider payment. Though probably desirable, such a reduction will not in itself solve Medicare's long-term problems; altering provider payment strategies might usefully be combined with the beneficiary payment model.

The Medicare insurance held by 83 percent of the elderly population generally reimburses providers according to a predetermined fee schedule. It pays on a per admission basis (the diagnostic related group, or DRG, system) for inpatient care, and it pays on a fee-for-service basis for physician care. In both cases, although hospitals and doctors in theory can refuse to accept these payment levels and thereby decline to treat Medicare beneficiaries, the great majority have not done so. Nevertheless, traditional Medicare is not governmental price-fixing, anathema to all economists who are believers in the virtue of markets. Instead, such a reimbursement policy is the expected behavior of a large insurer with a dominant market share. That the insurer happens to be administered (at several removes) by the government rather than a private firm makes little difference; a for-profit version of the Health Care Financing Administration with 83 percent of the high-use elderly market would behave much as the current Medicare program, though it might have less concern for the political ramifications of its managerial decisions. Even aggressive provisions, such as the refusal to reimburse the services of a physician for whom beneficiaries would be willing to pay extra or to pay for some services entirely on their own, are potentially useful methods of bargaining, since they channel more business to those physicians who do accept such terms.

Historically, traditional Medicare and private insurances have had one major difference. Private insurance was purchased in a competitive market; if some potential customers felt that an insurer was too aggressive—for example, by limiting the network of physicians through the kind of all-or-nothing payment provisions just described—those customers could switch to another, kinder insurer. But Medicare heavily subsidized just one insurer in most markets: the fee-for-service traditional Medicare plan with all its aggressive rules, limits on payment, criminal penalties, and slow reimbursement policies. This limitation was part of the bargain that we made with ourselves when Medicare was passed (or as time passed): to keep Medicare costs down, the desires of some better-off or more particular elders would have to be sacrificed at the altar of the good deal. The passage of Medicare+Choice, however, may have modified this bargain. According to this law, a private insurer can offer a plan that pays doctors more and receives a contribution from the Medicare program. (However, the premium for covered services is still constrained.) Of course, such an insurer would not start off with 83 percent of the Health Care Financing Administration's market share; we cannot be sure that the resulting competition will initially be a fair fight. However, the bureaucratic sluggishness and the political limits on traditional Medicare even up the odds. Explicit proposals to break up traditional Medicare's monopsony position have yet to be heard.

If traditional Medicare therefore retains this large market share, it could use its share to help contain costs further. The inpatient portion of

Medicare is already subject to what hospitals allege to be fairly strict payment limits, with annual updates proposed by the Medicare Advisory Commision's ProPac and its successor MedPAC in the zero-to-negative range. Hospital payment, I argue below, is largely a matter of choosing when and what volume of quality-improving but cost-increasing technology should be made available to beneficiaries. The recent controversy over Medicare's refusal to pay for lung-reduction surgery provides an excellent example of this. According to preliminary data, this new type of surgery appears to help patients with lung disease; expected health benefits are therefore positive. But there is a chance that there is no benefit. Conversely, expected (short-term) costs are positive, beyond a shadow of a doubt. Hence, Medicare has been calling for a delay in coverage until the positive effect is guaranteed. At present, no one has been willing to admit the obvious: the cost matters, and benefits, though positive, may not be worth the cost. The main problem is that Medicare has no method for judging what benefits are worth.

The situation with physician payment is much clearer. Medicare makes strenuous efforts to determine whether its payment policies are restricting access to physicians' services. And at present they are not. With only a few exceptions, physicians accept new and continuing Medicare patients. Surveys of beneficiaries find only tiny minorities of them reporting any problems with access. Those problems are primarily confined to the 7 percent of the Medicare population without Medicaid or Medigap coverage (generally low-income and disproportionately nonwhite), but even these problems show no sign of worsening. Although Medicare's payment schedule is below the fees that physicians post for their private fee-for-service patients, the eagerness of physicians to supply services to Medicare patients often means that those fee levels are above what physicians can collect for their private business from new private patients, most of whom are now covered by managed care or are unwilling to accept new services.

The supply of physicians' services under Medicare's current physician fee schedule is more than adequate. By implication, then, the fee schedule is too high. In the face of excess supply, an insurer concerned about its costs or its premiums should cut fees. It should continue to cut until some hints of access or shortage problems start to emerge. What it should do then depends on what trade-offs it is willing to make between access and costs. Medicare appears, at present and everywhere in the country, to be so far from that point that it need not make choices.

How much Medicare might save from a more aggressive payment

policy in the fee-for-service segment is hard to say. Physician reimbursements are important, especially in Part B, but, at about 40 percent of total Medicare payments, limits or slowdown in their rates of growth cannot do much good for the Part A trust fund and cannot save the system (although they could save the home health benefit recently transferred to Part B). However, even if not a panacea, payment rate cuts surely could help. Moreover, the part of Medicare operated by HCFA could extend this pricing power to a wider range of insurance products, with larger or different patterns of cost-sharing and coverage.

## Medicare and the Well-Off

While these steps might help improve Medicare, and might even stave off trust fund "bankruptcy" for a time, they do not really improve the efficiency of the financing and care delivery system. Instead, these changes shift costs—among different generations in the savings and investment scheme and to providers in the reimbursement scheme. I next focus on a scheme that can improve efficiency, although it may also engage in redistribution. This plan would reduce both the scope and the value of the Medicare benefit for higher-income or wealthy elderly. I have provided some technical arguments for and details on the scheme elsewhere (Pauly 1998).

The fundamental motivation for this type of change can be stated in several ways. The most common-sense explanation notes that the purpose of Medicare is to help elderly people obtain medical care that they cannot otherwise afford but that such help is not needed for moderate expenses for the moderately well-off or for all expenses for the rich. According to a more technical explanation, Medicare has caused some higher-income people to buy more medical insurance and medical care than they otherwise would, but this additional care does not represent needed consumption. My proposal would also redistribute income—a function that is more difficult to evaluate. The recently passed Medicare option of a medical savings account (MSA) does permit people to reduce their coverage somewhat, but it is peripheral to the overall Medicare program, and poorly designed. I propose a more comprehensive reform of Medicare benefits for the nonpoor, a reform that puts options for cost-limiting coverage at the center of the reform.

The general principle to be explored is this: the provision of health care that is both efficient and equitable to elders (as to the rest of the population) will require minimum coverage that varies inversely with income (decreases as income increases). By intuition, to obtain greater equality in the use of care, there must be greater *in*equality in the level of coverage. How much care and how much equality we desire are ultimately political value judgments. How much coverage is needed to achieve the amount of care regarded as desirable at each income level is ultimately a matter of empirical fact, and the data exist to make these estimates once the political process decides its goals.

Even without full implementation of this process, however, we can agree on some qualitative judgments. Very low-income people even at a moderate level of risk or very high risk people at a moderate level of income should have generous coverage. Very wealthy people at low risk, in contrast, can be expected to consume adequate amounts of care with little or no Medicare subsidy whatsoever. These people could be taken off Medicare; they would receive no subsidy but could choose whatever insurance they want.

Between these two extremes, efficiency and equity require subsidized insurance coverage, but such coverage can be partial. At incomes above but close to the poverty line, deductibles can remain low. At upper-middle-class income levels, the target or subsidized policy can be limited to a high-deductible catastrophic policy (although some might choose to buy more coverage on their own) with a small subsidy to match. The very rich would have no subsidy and no interference. In short, there should be income- and risk-related vouchers or subsidies: the insurance policies with which those subsidies must be used should have coverage requirements that decline with income.

## Why Change Medicare?

Medicare thus far has taken the classic social insurance form, providing the same nominal benefits to persons at all income levels, while financing those benefits with payroll taxes. In itself, uniformity of benefit is not necessarily objectionable. It avoids the need to determine the incomes or assets of elders, a process that can be both costly and distortionary, as the experience of the Medicaid nursing-home benefit implies. For some, an additional virtue of the social insurance form is that the benefit is politically supported by its middle-class recipients (and their children). It is not a "welfare benefit" for the undeserving poor, to be disparaged and depleted in periods of budgetary pressure or political confrontation, but a cherished right of the middle class, to be protected and strengthened.

Were the tax cost of furnishing such a Medicare subsidy likely to remain close to its initial nominal level, this argument might be accepted. Even though the Medicare program does cause some inefficiency, as shown below, it probably would not be challenged if it were perceived as affordable. However, the perception of affordability has surely vanished, both in the current period and in prospect.

The most conspicuous evidence of Medicare's problem concerns projections for the trust fund for the Part A benefit, hospitalization. Each year the trustees predict the date when this part of Medicare will be bankrupt. When the date nears, panic ensues; when, as in the current year, a combination of program changes and economic prosperity push the date back a few years, people are relieved.

But the potential "bankruptcy" of Medicare is not the real problem. Rather, the higher taxes needed to finance benefits (regardless of the state of the fictitious trust fund) are relevant. The trust fund records the collections of an earmarked payroll tax. As long as the sum of such collections (plus interest) exceeds the sum of benefits paid, the government can continue to pay these benefits with no increase in tax rates. When and if total disbursements equaled total collections to that point, the trust fund would have a zero balance. From that point onward, total spending per time period could not exceed the taxes collected per time period unless Congress permitted a "deficit," that is, unless general revenue tax collections supplemented the payroll taxes. (Using budgetary surpluses to shore up Medicare would effectively do this, but such a process is unlikely to be a permanent solution.)

It is not correct to say that Medicare Part A would "go bankrupt." At the point of zero balance, it would have zero assets but also zero current liabilities: it would be exactly *in balance*. It *is* correct to say that, henceforth, unless spending were controlled, taxes—either payroll taxes or general revenue taxes—would have to be raised. A trust fund balance of zero would have a strong signaling value; this is possibly one of the reasons why Medicare and Social Security used the earmarked tax–trust fund device. But the real economic issue occurs before bankruptcy and continues afterward if some fix other than reduced spending is used: the burden of and the economic distortion attributable to high tax rates persist.

**Taxes and Spending.** In an accounting sense, anything that reduces the growth of total spending will help assure the future of the Medicare trust fund. As table 4–1 indicates, the spending burden could be low-

TABLE 4–1

DISTRIBUTION OF THE ELDERLY BY FAMILY INCOME AS A
PERCENTAGE OF THE POVERTY LINE, 1968 AND 1997

| Family Income as a | Percentage of Population | |
|---|---|---|
| Percentage of Poverty Level | 1968 | 1997 |
| < 100 | 28.6 | 9.1 |
| < 200 | 34.3 | 30.6 |
| < 300 | 16.3 | 21.9 |
| < 400 | 9.3 | 13.9 |
| < 500 | 4.9 | 8.5 |
| > 500 | 6.6 | 15.9 |

SOURCE: Author's tabulation from the Current Population Survey.

ered now by considerably reducing or eliminating benefits to those elders with family incomes well in excess of the poverty line. About a quarter of those older than sixty-five now are in families with incomes above 400 percent of the poverty line, up from about 11 percent when Medicare was passed. Because these persons tend to be younger and in two-person families, we cannot translate their proportion of membership into a corresponding proportion of spending. Nevertheless, the basic message is crystal clear: in contrast to the situation when Medicare was passed, a sizable minority of beneficiaries now have incomes that are comfortably middle class and above. Even if only half of public spending on people who are over 400 percent of the poverty line could be reduced or shifted to beneficiaries, the tax burden could be substantially reduced. Such a change, if implemented now, would mean that rather than being wiped out in 2015, the Part A trust fund could continue a positive balance for at least another five years.

The relatively comfortable economic standing of today's elderly should not be overemphasized. The proportion with six-figure incomes is still tiny (though not the proportion with six-figure wealth). Only Social Security keeps many elderly families from slipping below the poverty line. Moreover, the relevant issue is the change in well-being of elders *relative to* that of wage earners. Still, no one can deny that many in the Medicare population now are more capable of paying for health benefits than when Medicare was passed, and that wage earners have not experienced anything close to this improvement. The Medicare deductible has modestly increased, as the Part B out-of-pocket payments have also. However, while the *proportion* of elderly income spent on medical care has remained roughly constant, the absolute *amount* of income available after medical expenses has surely increased on average; medical care has not come close to eating up the substantial growth in real income.

This recognition has already begun edging into the policy debate. A proposal for Medicare reform discussed in 1997 but not enacted would have had the very well off elderly pay either higher Part B premiums or higher cost-sharing. The income limit proposed was so high that the fiscal consequences would have been only symbolic. Current Social Security policy, which effectively taxes the benefits of higher income beneficiaries up to age seventy, is based on similar thinking.

**Rationales for Redistribution.** At one level, the argument for reducing Medicare's transfers to better-off elders is simple and powerful: they neither need nor deserve the help that they currently get, especially when their situation is evaluated relative to that of the average workers paying the payroll taxes. However, if the primary objective of reform is to generate a presumably fairer distribution of wealth, using Medicare reform to achieve this objective hardly seems to be the most direct route. More transparent alterations in the degree of progressivity of the income tax would be preferred. Indeed, a cynic (or a realist) might imagine that such additional redistribution in itself would be politically infeasible, because it would upset the prevailing political equilibrium, in which there does not seem to be a strong demand to soak the upper middle class further.

Two additional reasons beyond redistribution explain why reducing the flow of Medicare spending to better-off elders may be desirable. Both reasons concern efficiency. One reason deals with the efficient use of medical care. The other relates to the tax issue already raised.

The first argument is both fundamental and complex. The primary purpose of the Medicare program—clear from the original language— was to help seniors afford needed medical care. It was not intended to encourage saving, and it was not intended to protect bequests. The program therefore had two dimensions: to permit access to appropriate (neither deficient nor excessive) amounts of care and to protect seniors from the risk of unexpected out-of-pocket expenses that were large enough to affect their ability to obtain other important goods and services.

In considering first the behavior under the conventional or indemnity insurance currently chosen by 83 percent of elderly persons, there are two important empirical propositions. First, holding constant the illness level and all other influences on use, higher-income and more wealthy seniors will use more care and will spend more than others. Second, a given out-of-pocket expense is more easily budgeted the higher is the person's income.

The implications of these observations are profound. A single nominally uniform insurance policy produces distinctly nonuniform results. It causes all insureds to consume more care than if they were uninsured, but it produces higher levels of consumption by the well-off, compared with the levels of those with lower incomes. More precisely, if the level of coverage is chosen to ensure that lower-income beneficiaries consume needed care, this level must logically stimulate overconsumption by those with higher incomes. Conversely, if the level is set to induce appropriate consumption by the well-off, its coverage will be far too skimpy for lower-income families. Moreover, for many people of sufficiently high income and wealth, the level of consumption that they choose (possibly with private insurance) is probably adequate even without the Medicare subsidy; if the subsidy does anything, it induces them to consume more than adequate amounts of service.

The second issue relates to incentive effects of means-testing Medicare. If Medicare benefits are changed so that they depend inversely on income, this policy change has incentive effects on savings and work effort. While the burden and distortion of payroll taxes are reduced, a disincentive is now associated with what is effectively a tax on income and wealth once people become sixty-five. What is important for efficiency is the *net* excess burden, with a reduction in one distortion potentially offset by an increase in another.

The income-conditioning of Medicare benefits potentially affects two decisions. Most obviously, it affects the lifetime work effort, since it effectively taxes postretirement wealth. This effect may lead to a lower present value of lifetime total consumption; it may also lead to lower rates of saving (that is, a shift in lifetime consumption from postretirement to preretirement years) and a potential conversion of wealth to untaxed forms.

Most of the discussion of income-conditioned social insurance has dealt with Social Security rather than with Medicare, has been primarily conceptual rather than empirical, and has generally yielded a negative opinion about further means-testing of Social Security benefits (Neumark and Powers 1997). However, there are some important differences between Social Security and Medicare.

First, the value of Social Security benefits does increase with wage income, even if not proportionately. If workers foresee the effect of higher payroll taxes on their pensions, those taxes will deter their work effort less if—as for Medicare—no additional benefit is earned through higher wages. In contrast, a move from benefits that are positively related to income to those negatively related to income—as the introduction of means-testing for Social Security would do—is a much larger *increase* in the penalty on earning higher wages than means-testing for Medicare would be.

Second, Social Security pays benefits in money terms and, in this sense, is a close substitute for private savings. In contrast, Medicare, while providing a partial substitute for savings, furnishes a much less perfect one. As a result, a decrease in the expected benefit provided could lead to less of a savings offset.

Finally, the impact of means-testing either type of benefit on work effort is ambiguous. If earning a higher income now reduces the expected value of my Medicare benefit, will I work less because I am being punished for working and saving for a higher pension or annuity, or will I save more because I realize that I will need more savings to cover what Medicare does not? The random nature of the additional cost under Medicare leads to this ambiguity.

There is some empirical evidence that the availability of income-related benefits does reduce work effort (Neumark and Powers 1997). However, such effects, as noted, are not necessarily fatal flaws. The impact depends on how large they are. One strategy would be to offset many of the reduced health insurance benefits to the high-income population with increased Social Security payments. That approach, which would forgo much of the overall payroll tax savings but would retain the reduction in excessive medical care spending, does have some virtue.

**What to Adjust.** I have already sketched a way of tailoring the minimum Medicare benefit to income by varying the amount of required coverage. This is only one possible method. The more common approach, discussed during the Medicare reform debate, would raise Medicare Part B premiums for wealthy elders. A third alternative would be to postpone the age of Medicare eligibility for better-off seniors. Which is best?

The most common answer is that raising premiums is better than raising cost-sharing, because the former is easier to administer (Reischauer 1997). This is probably correct if Medicare is to be administered in its original single-insurer "defined benefits" form, which would require HCFA to adjust deductibles and coinsurance separately by income. However, there is an alternative: let the high-income beneficiary decide how to cope with a smaller subsidy. *Treat Medicare's payment as a defined contribution, and reduce both the contribution and the minimum required level of coverage for higher-income beneficiaries.* This procedure would be easier to administer, and the beneficiary could then be permitted to adjust (within limits) *either* by paying more to obtain coverage greater than the minimum *or* by accepting a policy with higher cost-sharing (or stronger managed care). It might even be possible to allow higher-income beneficiaries to choose to work for some years beyond age sixty-five and then to receive a more generous subsidy upon retirement.

**Some Design Issues.** Most analyses of income-based adjustments to the Medicare program have assumed that the basic coverage package would remain unchanged and that only the premium would be raised for higher-income beneficiaries. The few proposals to raise cost-sharing for higher-income beneficiaries implicitly assume that the premium would remain the same. In contrast, the proposal here is to change *both* the premium and the extent of coverage as incomes rise. The key decision from the viewpoint of efficiency is the minimum level of coverage; this level should fall as incomes rise.

If the actuarial value of coverage does decline as income rises, the premium required for this coverage might, beyond some income level, decline as well. At low-income levels, when the required level of coverage is high, the premium would have to be low and the tax-financed subsidy would have to be high. However, as incomes rise, the subsidy could fall, for two reasons: the required level of coverage declines and the beneficiary should be able to pay a larger fraction of the cost of that coverage. The larger the fraction of the premium paid by the beneficiary, the more likely the beneficiary will decline coverage. However, the experience of Medicare Part B shows that purchase is still nearly universal when the level of subsidy is as low as 70 percent of the premium. For instance, at some high-income level, people might be required to take coverage with an actuarial value half as great as current Medicare coverage, and they might be required to pay 70 percent of the premium for this coverage. Doing so would mean that the amount of tax-financed subsidy could be cut to 70 percent of half the current Medicare expense, or 35 percent of current spending. Such a design feature could further reduce the size of the subsidy needed.

# Medicare and Supplementation

Currently, the great majority of Medicare beneficiaries do not pay the deductibles and coinsurance. Most obtain private Medigap coverage; a smaller proportion of poor elders are dually eligible for Medicaid as well. This private supplementation causes two sorts of problems. First, Medigap coverage is generally expensive to administer; if a single insurer could manage the coverage, administrative costs could be lower. Second, Medigap coverage increases the use of the basic Medicare coverage, but the beneficiary is not charged for this. In this sense, Medigap is cross-subsidized. If this subsidy were curtailed, much supplementation might well disappear. (I return to this point below.)

But suppose, at some high-income level, the great majority of beneficiaries continued to purchase supplemental coverage entirely at their own expense. Such behavior signals that the subsidy to the basic coverage for this population is, at least at the margin, unnecessary and therefore excessive.

The technical argument here is complex because of two parameters to current, and potentially reformed, public policy: the size of the policy that must be purchased if any subsidy is to be paid and the size of the subsidy to buy that policy (that is, the difference between beneficiary premiums and the total actuarial cost for the policy). Efficiency depends primarily on the extent of coverage (and the associated rate of use of medical services); the subsidy induces people to buy any level of coverage and determines what they have available to spend on other things.

We can develop some easy conclusions about the extremes. Surely the income and wealth of some current beneficiaries are so great that they would, even without any Medicare coverage, buy as much care as they need. For them, no subsidy is necessary. At the other extreme, the income of some is so low that these beneficiaries will buy only needed care with the help of a fully subsidized Medicare policy; their income is also so low that they would never supplement this policy. Such elderly people with income near or below the poverty line are eligible for Medicaid coverage, which covers (often subject to reimbursement and other limits) the cost-sharing in Medicare and many services that Medicare does not cover. The most relevant and challenging group therefore is the set of elders with incomes just above the Medicaid eligibility limit. About 20 percent of the people in this income range ($10,000–15,000 in 1992) had no private supplementary insurance; this proportion is five times greater than for those with incomes between $35,000 and $50,000 (Chulis, Eppig, and Posail 1995).

The value judgment of society is most apparent here. Even though this group reports more problems in obtaining access than any other (even racial minorities or the disabled), society has shown no desire to provide them with more generous Medicare coverage. Perhaps the current level of unsupplemented Medicare coverage—with deductibles for Parts A and B, cost-sharing in both parts, and upper limits on coverage—is considered the socially adequate level of coverage for this population group. I do not agree with this judgment, but at the moment (and indeed for the past thirty years), this apparently represents the equilibrium of the political process regarding Medicare benefits.

This conclusion has an important implication. If Medicare coverage alone is socially adequate for people at the income level where supplementation is less common, it is certainly adequate for people with higher incomes, since those people will (other things being equal) surely use more care. It therefore follows that little or no social benefit is associated with the purchase of Medigap coverage for people with incomes above the Medicaid cutoff. However, since there is no social gain from supplementary coverage for these higher-income groups, their basic Medicare coverage could efficiently be less generous than it is, and the current level of subsidy for that coverage could be less. The objective here is to avoid subsidizing when the average level of use of care induced by subsidization has little or no social value at the margin. Subsidies therefore could be reduced. How might they be reduced, and what method would be best?

Reducing the level of the subsidized coverage is the best way to deal with those who can afford supplemental insurance. This reduction can be accomplished best by simultaneously reducing the size of the subsidy and the minimum levels of coverage. Upper-middle-income people could receive a smaller subsidy compared with today's Medicare but could still benefit from a subsidy even if they select policies with higher deductibles or stricter limits on services. They would not be *required* to take such limited coverage, but the size of the subsidy would be adjusted until the average person did not supplement.

This strategy, though logical, may seem draconian, precisely because it assumes that current Medicare-only coverage is adequate. An alternative approach would retain current Medicare coverage limits and would reduce the subsidy (raise the Medicare enrollee premium) until the level of supplemental coverage fell enough that the overall level of coverage (basic Medicare plus Medigap) was regarded as adequate.

## Policies and Planning

That strategy argues for required coverage that would vary by income level and for no encouragement to supplementing that coverage. Yet, many experts find an attractive alternative in offering a uniform "basic" coverage to all, with supplementation entirely at the individual consumer's expense. At the allocative efficiency level, as long as the basic coverage were optimal for the lowest-income users, one might argue that no harm comes from providing the same level of the social good to all others. If others accept this level of provision and do supplement it with their own money, the result is still efficient unless, for some reason, higher-income people are to be discriminated against.

There is a distributional difference from the income-conditioned scheme, but no efficiency difference. Besides, the uniform benefit means that income does not have to be measured again for the recipients and that the overall tax system can be adjusted to whatever is equitable. Why bother with any program-specific adjustment to benefits?

This argument would be persuasive for a social good that gave the same amount of resources to all users. However, as noted, the same nominal health insurance coverage or policy does not yield equality of resource use or service consumption regardless of income. The better-off get more out of a given nominal policy than the less well off. Indeed, for everyone to use the same amount of resources and the same amount of care, *different* policies should be offered to people at different income levels.

Would the program work differently if the basic coverage were managed care? Research is less definitive here, but there is much evidence that higher-income people obtain more services even under systems that are rationed on the supply side. It is not so much income per se, but the higher education that usually accompanies it, which allows the better-off to talk their way around treatment protocols and financial incentives to doctors. From the British National Health Service to Hometown HMO, use is not equal; the more affluent get more, other things being equal. There may be *less* income-related inequality under managed care than under fee-for-service, but there will surely be some substantial amount of it (Nelson et al. 1998). Just as before, coverage must be less equal if results are to be more equal. Moreover, whatever happens *within* a managed-care plan, the well-off can, and do, buy more generous versions of such plans, whether generosity is measured by the size of the network, the permissiveness of clinical pathways, or the presence of an easy point-of-service (POS) option.

There is an important qualification to the no-subsidy-for-supplementation rule. Subsidies must necessarily be uniform for broad classes of individuals. Suppose that an income category needs a subsidy to induce the average person (with average tastes) to choose the appropriate level of coverage without supplementation. A minority of persons in that category, probably the most risk-averse, might choose to supplement. Permitting such behavior (rather than "custom tailoring" a subsidy scheme) is probably prudent. After all, the alternative—identifying the risk-averse beforehand as candidates for smaller subsidies— is neither practical nor politically attractive.

If almost all persons in some category supplement a subsidized policy, the subsidy must be too great (or the chosen policy must be too stingy). Either way, something is not right.

## Where Are We Going—and How Do We Get There?

Discussions of income-conditioning Medicare benefits have been decidedly low-key and small-scale. The proposals considered so far have involved limiting the impacts to Part B premiums for the highest-income groups, with consequent fiscal impacts that are more symbolic than substantial (Moon and Kuntz 1996). I have argued for a more thorough revision of Medicare based on income adjustment, a change substantial enough to achieve some fiscal good. In this section I consider two apparently contradictory ideas: some small steps in the direction of income-conditioning that could allow us to experiment with the idea and some arguments that income-conditioning, if fully implemented, would lead to a radical reform of the Medicare program and of health care.

Fundamentally, we should consider restructuring the way Medicare treats older people who are not poor, because the program cannot afford to continue as it has treated them: funding coverage acceptable to middle-class seniors largely through taxes imposed on the rest of the population. Some parts of Medicare—insurance coverage that provides access to needed care—are most definitely worth preserving, but these components are at risk from the growing cost of paying for the other parts that are less essential. Low-income elders need comprehensive insurance coverage that is more generous than current Medicare; high-income elders need catastrophic coverage at a reasonable price; and middle-class people of all ages need moderate taxes. One way to preserve these three objectives is to make a bargain with those elders lucky enough to be moderately well-off: in return for smaller government subsidies for them and for lower taxes on their children, they would have more freedom to select insurance. Most especially, they would be allowed to choose how their health care spending would be controlled (and, indeed, whether it were to be controlled at all). They may choose out-of-pocket payments at the point of use; managed care with strict protocols, low reimbursement rates to providers, and financing incentives to providers to be frugal; or no limits at all—and then reap the gains or pay the costs of choosing these options.

For the very rich, subsidies can be ended and freedom made unlimited. For the majority in the middle class and above, the virtually obligatory, collectively controlled insurance will be available, but only as an option or a foundation for protection against truly catastrophic expenses. This group can pay for more themselves—from savings accounts, by reduced current consumption, or by additional premiums—and can choose whether to receive experimental treatments, whether to pay doctors whatever they charge, and whether care will be managed. However, for lower-income beneficiaries, even those too rich for Medicaid, coverage will be fairly generous, because catastrophic coverage will be inefficiently low.

Although immediate and aggressive income-conditioning would maximize Medicare's fiscal health, that step may be neither politically feasible nor fair to current beneficiaries. Some modifications of the current policy could be made now. These changes could include raising premiums for Part B for the well-off, permitting better-off seniors greater use of catastrophic health insurance, with or without medical savings accounts, and, more generally, allowing people at higher-income levels to convert Medicare into an explicit defined contribution. In contrast, allowing low-income elders to have medical savings accounts and catastrophic coverage would probably be inefficient. An announced schedule of reductions in subsidies would permit the near-elderly to adjust their savings and insurance-purchasing behavior now so that the transition at age sixty-five would be less disruptive. Assuring low-income seniors that their benefits are not at risk would lead to a reduction in worry and opposition.

I have even argued elsewhere (Pauly 1998) that, in the broadest perspective, nothing justifies Medicare's existence as a separate public program if the rest of the population could be enrolled in a universal health insurance program financed by income- and risk-adjusted predetermined credits. A larger proportion of older people would receive increased credits because of chronic illness, but no distinction would be necessary between people with serious illnesses because of their age. A design issue is whether the credit should increase with age, independent of diagnosed chronic conditions; this social judgment actually means relatively little, because the increase in premiums for the healthy as they age is quite gradual and is usually matched with growing income and wealth.

**Objectives and Limits.** Without any additional changes, the Medicare Part A trust fund is expected to reach a zero balance about 2015. More seriously from an economic perspective, the implied payroll tax rate to support both Parts A and B of Medicare is expected to double or triple from its current 4.2 percent level by about 2025; added to a somewhat higher rate of Social Security tax, the implicit rate to support social insurance would range from 22 to 33 percent.

Obviously the contribution income-conditioning Medicare would make to improving this situation depends on the degree of that policy change. While the growth in the number and proportion of nonpoor elderly has been striking both in itself and relative to changes in the distribution of income among workers, there may still not be enough rich elderly whose additional payments could substantially reduce the system's problem. Conversely, the alternative of cutting benefits or raising premiums for all or virtually all beneficiaries is difficult to support, since it appears to contradict the purposes of Medicare and Social Security. For income-conditioning to help appreciably, the more numerous upper-middle class would have to bear the burden. In this section I present some calculations intended to sketch a serious program of income-conditioning and its effects.

Recent proposals to have the well-off pay more are generally too limited to have more than a symbolic effect, especially with a focus on Part B premiums and on contributions as a proportion of Part B benefits. True, all beneficiaries pay premiums for the nominally voluntary Part B (supplemental) insurance, and these benefits are heavily subsidized out of general revenue taxes paid by the entire population, at a much higher rate than originally planned (currently at about 75 percent compared with the original 50-50 financing). In contrast, the substantially larger Part A is funded by an earmarked payroll tax. The average current retiree did not and does not pay anything near the full cost of either his Part A or Part B coverage. Conversely, a high-income, high-wage retiree probably did pay more taxes over his lifetime than the actuarial expected value of his Part A and Part B benefits. I do not distinguish much, then, between the nominal funding of the two parts but rely on substitution in taxation and fungibility in the budget to justify this treatment.

Substantially increasing the proportion of Part B premiums paid by the very well-off (say, to 75 percent of the premium rather than the current 25 percent) would not raise much extra money or reduce taxes much. Moon and Kuntz (1996) estimate that beginning to increase premiums for those singles with incomes of $50,000 and couples with incomes of $75,000, up to 75 percent of Part B premiums, would raise amounts equal to only 0.6 percent of total Medicare spending. Despite a 6 percent increase in Part B premium revenue, that revenue accounts for slightly less than 10 percent of total Medicare benefits; its impact on the overall cost of Medicare is small. Such an increase would permit a tax reduction of about 0.5 percent.

With total benefits held constant and with increases only to Part B premiums, such increases would have to apply to virtually all the Medicare population to be noticeable. The largest increase simulated by Moon and Kuntz would permit only about a 3 percent reduction in taxes and would raise all Part B premiums up to 30 percent of costs (from 25 percent) and then up to 100 percent of costs at incomes levels of $75,000 and $110,000 for singles and couples, respectively.

## Solutions, Anyone?

These calculations suggest that relatively small steps will not contribute much toward solving the problem. However, applying income-conditioning to Part A as well as to Part B, by adjusting the value of the Medicare contribution with income as I have suggested, could do more. A program of income adjustment for Part A similar to Moon and Kuntz's largest increase could reduce Medicare spending by about 8 percent, approximately the current gap between spending and tax collections.

The problem with Medicare's future is not primarily the mismatch of a growing elderly population and a shrinking payroll tax base. The elderly population grows at 2 percent per year; the number of workers grows at 0.8 percent per year; and real wages per worker might, with some luck, grow at the 1.2 percent per year needed to make the growth in the payroll tax base equal the growth in the number of seniors.

The real problem is the estimated *growth* in real spending per beneficiary. As Victor Fuchs (1998) has recently shown, even the somewhat lower growth targets following the Balanced Budget Act lead to projections of increases in Medicare spending relative to beneficiary income from the current level of about 15 percent to 50 percent or more.

Income-conditioning of premiums and coverage may still offer a way out. We can think of the solutions as having two parts, both painful but both possible. Income-related premiums could cover the current and near-future shortfalls in the Medicare program. Doing so would increase premiums for the well-off above the level of Part B spending (about $2,000 per beneficiary) but well below the total of $5,000. The second part is more radical: if current workers retire with relatively high incomes and wealth, they must finance their own consumption of costly but beneficial *new* technology. New technology, not rising provider incomes or growing waste, causes the projected spending growth. If the one-quarter to one-third of beneficiaries who are well-off would fund their own use of such technology, the growth rate in spending per beneficiary could be cut by the same proportion. Putting the two pieces together, we could cut the growth in the Medicare tax rate in half. The range of payroll taxes for Medicare and Social Security in 2030 would fall from 22–30 percent to 19–22 percent. Though not perfect, this radical solution may be as good as we can get. When combined with provider payment restraint and advanced funding, it may permit a tolerable outcome.

In health insurance, as in most other aspects of life, we do not want to make the perfect but unattainable the enemy of the good and feasible. We cannot afford to provide seniors (or the rest of the population) with all the medical care that they want, but we can afford to provide them with the care that they need.

# References

Chulis, G. S., F. J. Eppig, and J. A. Poisal. 1995. "Ownership and Average Premiums for Medicare Supplementary Insurance Policies." *Health Care Financing Review* 17(1) (fall): 255–75.

Fuchs, V. 1998. "'Provide, Provide'—The Economics of Aging." Paper presented at Texas A&M conference, "Medicare Reform: Issues and Answers," April 3.

Gramm, P., A. Rettenmaier, and T. Saving. 1998. "Medicare Policy for Future Generations—Search for a Permanent Solution." *New England Journal of Medicine* 338 (April 30): 1307–10.

Moon, M., and C. Kuntz. 1996. "Increasing Medicare's Part B Premium." *1996 Commonwealth Fund Report.*

Nelson, L., R. Brown, M. Gold, A. Ciemenecki, and E. Docteur. 1998. "Access to Care in Medicare HMO's, 1996." In *Contemporary Managed Care*, edited by M. Gold. Chicago: Health Administration Press.

Neumark, D., and E. Powers. 1997. "Means Testing Social Security." PRC WP 17-24, Pension Research Council, Philadelphia.

Pauly, M. V. 1998. "Should Medicare Be Less Generous to Higher Income Beneficiaries?" Paper presented at Texas A&M conference, "Medicare Reform: Issues and Answers," April 3.

Reischauer, R. D. 1997. "Midnight Follies." *Washington Post*, June 22, p. C7.

# 5

## Managing the Medicare Insurance Market

### Len M. Nichols

M edicare is our most sacred social contract precisely because it binds generations of Americans together with promises kept. It has achieved much success in lengthening and improving the quality of life for senior citizens since 1965, when it was implemented over the strenuous objections of powerful groups that now claim to support the goals of the program. While accomplishing these impressive feats, Medicare has become both our most popular public program and a program in need of structural repair, for it has developed some serious imbalances. Without repair, it may not be able to serve us as well in the twenty-first century. This chapter presents an approach to that repair that seeks to preserve our collective commitment to quality health care for all elderly.

I am grateful to Marilyn Moon of the Urban Institute and to Bob Helms, the editor of this volume, for helpful comments on an earlier draft. I remain responsible for all errors. The opinions expressed are my own and do not necessarily reflect the views of the Urban Institute, its trustees, or its sponsors.

The current policy discussion about restructuring Medicare is really a question about how to channel market forces to serve both Medicare beneficiaries and taxpayers. Sadly, the process is not as simple as setting the market absolutely free; completely unregulated health insurance markets have not performed well for the elderly, and there is little reason to be optimistic about laissez faire now. All insurance markets need a few structural safeguards to work well for anyone other than the continuously healthy.

But with those safeguards, which I outline below, modern insurance markets can work well. While we must be careful, harnessing the tremendous power of a well-structured private market to serve the Medicare program may be the best way to achieve acceptable trade-offs among our long-run goals of quality, choice, and an affordable public price tag. When coupled with reasonable financing and program flexibility over time, Medicare should remain a bedrock commitment on which all Americans can depend.

## The Evident Imbalances

There are two fundamental problems of the current Medicare program: (1) the inflation-adjusted cost per beneficiary is growing at an unsustainable rate, more than 5 percent per year for the past twenty-five years, and (2) the ratio of beneficiaries to workers will increase precipitously as the baby boomers begin to retire after 2010. The baby boomer problem cannot be properly addressed until the cost-growth problem is solved. All solutions to Medicare's fundamental problems, those described in this volume and elsewhere, require reductions in the real growth rate of cost per beneficiary.

A little algebra will make the stark nature of this challenge clear.[1] Let $B$ equal the number of elderly beneficiaries, $c$ equal the expected costs of covered health service per beneficiary, $p$ equal the fraction of those costs paid for by beneficiaries through premium payments, $w$ equal the average earnings of workers, $L$ equal the number of workers in society, and $t$ equal the payroll tax rate required to finance the pay-as-you-go Medicare program. In equilibrium, program costs are completely financed by beneficiaries and taxes:

$$cB = pcB + twL. \qquad (5\text{--}1)$$

Now the total population $(T)$ is divided into the share that is young $(y)$, who are not eligible for Medicare, and the nonyoung $(1 - y)$, who are. Only some fraction of the young ($f$) work. Therefore $L = fyT$, and $B = (1-y)T$. Substitution into equation 1 and solving for $t$, the required payroll tax rate, yield

$$t = [(1-p)c/w][(1-y)/fy].    (5-2)$$

The first bracketed term represents the publicly financed Medicare costs per dollar of wages, and the second term is the ratio of beneficiaries to workers. The required tax rate increases with both ratios. Health policy can affect only two of the five key parameters in our pay-as-you-go tax rate equation: $p$, the fraction of Medicare costs that beneficiaries are asked to pay in premiums, and $c$, the average covered cost per beneficiary.

As society ages, $y$ will continue to decline. Unless labor force participation increases enough to offset this, $fy$ will continue on its current downward path (as for most member-countries of the Organization for Economic Cooperation and Development, OECD, and some developing countries as well). Then one or more of three things must happen: (1) growth in the cost per beneficiary must be curtailed; (2) the fraction of covered health costs borne by the elderly and their families must increase; and (3) the payroll tax rate must increase. Clearly, the more success we have with the first, the less pain we must inflict with the other two actions.

To illustrate the order of magnitude of this problem, if we hold $p$ constant at today's level (9.8 percent) and current growth trends continue for all variables on the right-hand side of equation 5–2, the required payroll tax rate, $t$, will increase from today's implicit 5.5 percent to 14.4 percent in the next twenty years.[2] A doubling of the current beneficiary share, $p$, only reduces the required tax rate in 2018 to 13.2 percent. Given the nature of the political discourse over the past few years, it is hard to imagine that double-digit payroll tax rates for Medicare alone will ever be politically acceptable.

Reducing annual real growth in costs per beneficiary from the historical 5 percent to the currently projected 3 percent and doubling the beneficiary share would bring the required payroll tax rate down to 8.9 percent by 2018. As a final example, if we could somehow reduce the annual real growth of costs per beneficiary to 1 percent, then we could keep $p$ on its current trajectory to 12 percent, and the payroll tax rate would have to rise to a level no higher than 6.6 percent.

Some payroll tax increase is inevitable and reasonable to expect as the share of the population older than sixty-five increases in the first half of the twenty-first century. Controlling the growth rate of costs per beneficiary is the key to minimizing that tax increase, which will surely remain a goal even as we preserve our commitment to all elderly. This chapter focuses on politically palatable ways to reduce the growth in $c$, the Medicare-covered health services cost per beneficiary.

*Palatable* means preserving equitable access to health care of acceptable quality for all seniors. The implicit assumption in this chapter is that $c$ is growing faster within the current structure of Medicare than is required to accomplish our goals. If this assumption, though shared by many policy analysts today, turns out to be false, then the intergenerational problems in the next century will be even more difficult politically than they now appear.

## The General Solution

The practical goal of long-term structural reform of Medicare is to make the competition for next-generation managed-care and health insurance plans work well. By *next-generation*, I mean health plans that deliver and provide proof of high-quality processes and outcomes for beneficiaries who use that information to make informed choices about specific health plan and health provider arrangements. By *competition*, I mean market competition among a variety of arrangements, including not just health maintenance organizations (HMOs) and point-of-service (POS) plans, but also preferred provider organizations (PPOs), provider-sponsored organizations (PSOs), and even private indemnity plans. By *work well*, I mean provide good quality care for all beneficiaries, offer a reasonable choice of plans and providers, and do this at acceptable social resource cost. Aligning Medicare with appropriately managed market forces is essential for simultaneous realization of all these goals.

Accountability is the key to making any market work. Buyers need to be able to evaluate what they are getting, and sellers need to be forced by competition to produce quality products efficiently and to provide enough information for evaluation of the quality of the product or service itself. While much analytical attention has focused on the inefficiencies resulting from Medicare's many complex pricing rules, the absence of reporting requirements and accountability for Medicare risk plans is at least as serious an impediment to better value for the taxpayers' dollars in the near term. The purchasing arrangements for private and public health insurance that are working well today all focus on making health plans and providers accountable to the buyer and patients in ways that facilitate value-based purchasing.

*Value-based purchasing* is more than a consultant's buzzword, although it is surely also that. It means getting what a person pays for or demanding to know why not and then taking remedial action—including perhaps switching providers—on the basis of that knowledge.

Successful principles for health insurance–purchasing systems today are being practiced by groups as diverse as the San Francisco–based Pacific Business Group on Health; the Minnesota Buyers Health Care Action Group; the Colorado Health Care Purchasing Alliance in Denver; the Employer Health Care Alliance Cooperative of Madison, Wisconsin; the California Health Insurance Purchasing Cooperative; the Washington State Health Care Authority; and the Federal Employees Health Benefits Program (FEHBP). More than 100 business coalitions for purchasing health insurance have sprung up in recent years. Most successful examples are practicing rather similar variants of the principles of managed competition to demand and get health plan accountability (Meyer et al. 1997; Enthoven and Singer 1996; Maxwell et al. 1998; Feldman and Dowd 1998; Robinson and Powers 1998).

There are many differences in detail and even philosophy. But the real-world experience of employers and state governments suggests six important steps to implement value-based purchasing of health insurance. The next sections examine these steps and make recommendations for each of them in the context of creating a twenty-first-century health insurance market for Medicare beneficiaries.

## A Preliminary Caveat

Before we get to the precise details, an important clarification of what we can and cannot do quickly is in order. Medicare is a large, complex program serving 39 million beneficiaries in every state and the District of Columbia. Four million of these are older than eighty-five, and almost 5 million are disabled (HCFA 1997). Approximately 16 percent are also enrolled in Medicaid, and almost two-thirds of Medicare beneficiaries live in households with incomes below $20,000. Unlike the nonelderly insured through employer plans, 87 percent of Medicare beneficiaries are still in the fee-for-service (FFS) part of the program. For these and other reasons, managing competition to work well for Medicare beneficiaries is different and may be harder, at least at first, than for the employed population younger than sixty-five. These facts alone should encourage a sequencing of modest goals rather than the disruption of thrusting all the elderly into the individual health insurance marketplace.

Few managed-care plans know how to make money caring for the chronically ill and disabled elderly and are therefore skittish. Most states have not put their populations receiving supplemental security income (SSI) into Medicaid managed care nearly as quickly as the mothers and children in the Aid to Families with Dependent Children (AFDC) or in the Temporary Assistance for Needy Families (TANF) program. Congress must understand—as the Health Care Financing Administration (HCFA) and the providers who serve this population surely do—that transitions out of Medicare FFS will be slower and more painful for the chronically ill; therefore FFS must be preserved for the foreseeable future. Furthermore, about a quarter of Medicare beneficiaries live in rural areas where managed care is not available. Some areas may never realize effective competition among health plans.

The harder question that must be addressed before the reform process can be appropriately focused is this: Should FFS Medicare be required to compete like other health plans, or should it be kept primarily as a fallback for those who are not yet ready for the brave new world of competition? Some analysts have concluded that the long-run gains in efficiency from forcing real competition between traditional FFS and private managed-care plans would outweigh the short-run transition costs of the most vulnerable Medicare populations (Butler and Moffit 1995; Feldman and Dowd 1998).

Perhaps I am in less of a hurry to get the government out of the FFS business than they are. Perhaps I am more worried about selection effects mitigating competition between FFS and managed-care plans. I am not confident of our ability to measure the emotional costs and downside risks of choosing a health plan for the first time in a world of information overload, a world in which chronically ill beneficiaries know exactly how hard it was to find the providers with whom they are now comfortable (Jones 1998) and in which beneficiaries have little real hope of acquiring the detailed comparative information needed for informed decisions for at least three to five years.

Even if we could measure these costs accurately and weigh them fairly against plausible estimates of efficiency gains from forcing this kind of competition, structural reform discussions should keep in mind that the next two years already present many potentially sweeping changes to beneficiaries. Despite all the 1997 Balanced Budget Act (BBA) discussions about providing more choices and opening up Medicare to many different types of health plans, the fact that some carriers reduced their service areas or dropped out of the Medicare program altogether for 1999 is the first unsettling manifestation that many beneficiaries have seen of the new world of health plan competition. Still, BBA was enacted, and thus the full range of Medicare+Choice plans could enter the Medicare marketplace all over the country in the next two years (there appear to be fewer new types of plans—PPOs, PSOs— than expected when the BBA passed). As many as seven competitive bidding demonstrations will be getting under way in the next three years. Medicare+Choice and the new risk-adjustment mechanism that will be implemented in 2000 will change the risk-contracting portion of Medicare so much that it is highly unlikely that FFS Medicare could simultaneously compete and serve as a backup for disabled and other beneficiaries. Some of these beneficiaries might be reluctant, understandably, to enter managed-care plans only one year after the high-decibel rhetoric and federal attention devoted to creating new "patient rights" vis-à-vis managed-care plans.

It seems wiser and much safer to let the new Medicare+Choice plans assimilate into beneficiaries' consciousness while we learn what we can from the competitive bidding demonstrations and the new risk-adjustment experiences. We should also conduct demonstrations to see if specific disease-management or functional-status case-management programs might be a cost-effective way to provide high-quality and cost-effective managed care to the chronically or seriously ill. In the meantime, FFS Medicare should modernize and transform itself into what it will most likely become: a giant PPO with extensive provider-reporting requirements and utilization-management techniques.

But to throw FFS Medicare into the marketplace before we have improved our risk adjusters or FFS utilization-management techniques is to kill FFS Medicare knowingly as an option for all because of adverse selection. Undoubtedly, the sickest Medicare beneficiaries would disproportionately remain in FFS. Imperfect risk adjusters would therefore force the FFS "premium bid" to be much higher than that for managed-care plans; this result would only worsen the selection disadvantages of FFS Medicare in the short run. Five to seven years from now, FFS Medicare should be much better able to compete, and at that time a determination can be made about whether it should become more like a giant self-funded PPO for all or a safety net for those whom risk-bearing managed-care plans may never serve well (risk adjusters may never make plans truly indifferent about enrolling chronically ill beneficiaries and keeping them satisfied with their care).

The remainder of this chapter emphasizes managing the competition among risk-bearing plans outside FFS Medicare, with FFS remaining an option for beneficiaries at the out-of-pocket price of the Part B premium (or the $p$ equivalent from the equations above, if we manage to abolish the arbitrary distinctions between the parts of Medicare). While retaining the FFS option complicates the competition among the plans somewhat, it also serves as an essential safeguard against experimentation gone awry and as a constraint with implications that can be analyzed rather than as a wrongheaded mistake to lament and assume away.

## Insurance Market Management Techniques

In what follows, I assume that HCFA retains the statutory right to remain the sole purchasing agent for Medicare beneficiaries but also will be given the authority to delegate that power to local private agents (for example, employers on behalf of their retirees, nonprofit corporations), while the agency retains oversight and ultimate responsibility to Congress. I also assume that the payment system for Medicare+Choice based on adjusted average per capita costs (AAPCC) will be jettisoned as soon as the competitive bidding experiments have been evaluated, so that some form of competitive bidding becomes the framework of Medicare's insurance purchasing.

**Step 1: Define Benefit Packages.** Supporters of managed competition have long advocated standard benefit packages to enable consumers to comparison shop among plans and eliminate risk selection by benefit design (a time-honored technique of insurers). Some analysts, focused on the welfare losses from an imperfect match between defined benefits and individual preferences, argue against standard benefit requirements (Butler and Moffit 1995; Dowd, Feldman, and Christianson 1996; Feldman and Dowd 1998). Most advanced practitioners of value-based insurance purchasing employ standard benefit packages; FEHBP is one of the most prominent that does not.

The issue boils down to a trade-off. Unfettered benefit-design options would likely have two effects: insurers could make higher profits (or they would not be offered) and more consumers could find a package more consistent with their perceived individual needs. But the transactions costs of benefit design prevent all possible benefit configurations from being offered (Newhouse 1996); there will still be some welfare losses, and these losses could be substantial for the higher-risk beneficiaries whom insurers do not want to attract. Widely varying packages would enable profit-seeking insurers to accomplish additional risk segmentation; some benefits would have high prices, not because of the actuarial costs of the specific services, but because of the expected risk selection that those benefits would engender. Some who would select parsimonious packages may be quite disappointed to learn that they did not anticipate their full range of uncertain health care needs each year.

Two specific experiences support the majority vote of organized purchasers and recommend standard benefit packages. One is that of CalPERS, the California public employees retirement system, which was among the first to practice managed-competition principles. CalPERS began without standard benefit packages but soon switched to them to enhance comparison shopping and to reduce selection effects (Robinson and Powers 1998).

The other example is the experience of Medicare beneficiaries with the Medigap market. Under laissez faire, insurers exploited the abundant confusion to select risks and to sell duplicative policies to many seniors. The Baucus amendments of 1980 called for voluntary industry standards, but seniors still observed literally hundreds of Medigap policy configurations and found it quite difficult to compare the plans. The Omnibus Budget Reconciliation Act of 1990 (OBRA) addressed this shortcoming by specifying ten distinct types of Medigap policies. The vast majority of market participants think that the Medigap market is functioning much better now than before the benefit standardization reforms (Rice, Graham, and Fox 1997). States, by the way, administer these Medigap regulations under broad HCFA guidelines and oversight.

My judgment that standard benefit packages would strengthen the Medicare insurance market does not mean that I support a one-size-fits-all benefits package. There should be at least two distinct cost-sharing options and a few specific supplemental service packages, but they too must be defined to keep competition focused on the twin dimensions of price and quality, and not risk selection. These supplements could be thought of as building blocks, with reduced cost-sharing to start and then prescription drugs, dental, vision, etc., added until a fully comprehensive policy emerged. Additional beneficiary premiums (beyond the Part B, or $p$, obligation) would likely be necessary for at least some packages.

Three additional questions merit attention. What packages do insurers bid on? Should the same package be offered everywhere? How should we treat Medigap-only insurers?

Medicare is a public program with a statutory benefit package for all beneficiaries regardless of their state of residence. The current package is less generous than most private plans for garden-variety acute care: it does not have an out-of-pocket maximum or cover prescription drugs. Partly because of favorable selection and partly because of efficiencies, more than 60 percent of current Medicare HMOs offer beneficiaries benefits well beyond the standard package at no extra premium cost. Plans offer extra benefits because Medicare rules prevent them from offering cash rebates to beneficiaries. These zero-premium benefits vary with the current AAPCC distribution. In exchange for the Medicare payment to health plans, different Medicare beneficiaries receive different benefits—based partly on where they live—beyond the parsimonious basic package. Thus, the current system is inequitable.

These facts suggest three principles for benefit-package specification that would minimize disruption and beneficiaries' confusion and would maximize the benefits of competitive bidding. First, plans should submit bids on the basic package, as well as indicate their marginal charge to a beneficiary of average risk on all defined supplemental policies that they want to offer. Such bids would reveal to the government the full implications for beneficiary premiums of setting the government payment at any particular level or according to a formula based on the distribution of received bids. (Step 5 elaborates on setting the government payment.)

Second, Medicare should not try to force all zero-premium supplemental benefits to be the same everywhere. Some or all of the defined benefit supplements (above the basic and the cost-sharing reductions) could be allowed to vary by locality; these bidding processes would also be administered locally. GM manages to tailor its health plan offerings to local conditions in multiple states and countries; HCFA in some ways does so now through the zero-premium benefit determinations. Supplementary offerings could then reflect local differences in delivery costs or beneficiary preferences.

The relative parsimony of the Medicare benefit package created the Medigap industry, which has ballooned as more than two-thirds of all beneficiaries have either individually purchased or employer-sponsored Medigap coverage. Medigap coverage plays a useful role for beneficiaries who are worried about large out-of-pocket obligations for hospitalization or other serious episodes. However, the comprehensiveness of many Medigap policies has clearly increased the costs of the overall Medicare program, as lower cost-sharing increases the use of basic services. This effect is problematic if Medigap-only vendors are allowed to offer supplements that would be used in conjunction with private

Medicare+Choice plans, which are responsible for delivering those basic services.

There are two solutions to this problem. With new statutory authority, HCFA could force Medigap insurers to offer the basic package (this requirement would result in proper pricing of the supplements, because the insurers would have to internalize the moral hazard costs that they impose on the basic plan). Or HCFA could restrict Medicare+Choice enrollees to purchasing supplements only from vendors of their own basic plans or from other Medicare+Choice vendors. The former solution is preferred, for it would realign the supplemental prices vis-à-vis Medicare FFS as well, but it is also not likely to survive the interest-group lobbies. The latter choice would at least protect Medicare+Choice plans and allow competition among them to be untainted by Medigap insurers.

**Step 2: Define Enrollment and Marketing Rules.** Annual open enrollment, with no plan-switching between those periods, would clearly reduce some adverse selection that FFS Medicare suffers vis-à-vis risk-contract HMOs at present, with the thirty-day disenrollment policy. Annual enrollment is palatable only if there is an agreed external review process that HCFA enforces in a timely manner. Virtually all successful purchasers of health insurance use an annual enrollment period, and no one seems inclined to shorten or lengthen it.

Private firms have an interest and a right to present themselves in a favorable light to potential beneficiaries. This interest and right, however, are complemented and perhaps counterbalanced by HCFA's obligation to ensure that all Medicare beneficiaries are treated fairly and are aware of all choices and of the implications of those choices.

HCFA's preparation and dissemination of comparative plan information (discussed in step 3) are crucial here. This information would likely be perceived as a buyer's guide. HCFA must approve all marketing materials and recruitment techniques to ensure basic accuracy so that beneficiaries will not be confused by industry advertising.

Some prefer little or no role for government here. Private groups should be allowed to produce their own plan and provider rankings, much as the *Washington Checkbook Guide* rates FEHBP plans. But the special case of potentially frail Medicare beneficiaries, with their entitlement to services and our moral commitment to them, argues for thorough government oversight of marketing and enrollment as well as direct governmental provision of objective comparative information, at least until the private market can generate such information itself. Even then, because of low-income beneficiaries and for free-rider concerns (since information is a public good, the private market is likely to undersupply it), government should always be involved in dissemination.

**Step 3: Collect and Disseminate Enough Information to Inform Enrollees about Comparative Quality Measures and to Facilitate Plan or Provider Switching.** Health plan reporting is a prerequisite for the evaluation of quality outcomes, a key component to next-generation managed care and all successful health delivery systems of the twenty-first century. Without a foundation of quality reporting and assessment, no market-based purchasing strategy can ever perform well. True accountability means timely auditable data on measures that matter to patients. Most successful private buyers require and receive data that guide consumer actions and employer-sponsor negotiations with plans and provider groups.

Definitive measures of outcomes adjusted by case mix, especially for ambulatory care, will likely never be perfect. All participants should be diligent and cautious in making irrevocable judgments based on the available measures. Progress has been made in developing measures that are likely to be correlated with true outcome quality: the case for waiting until better measures come along weakens every day. At a minimum, statistics about basic use should be available as soon as possible. The sooner the reporting of use data is a requirement, the sooner even more constructive data will be forthcoming as a natural and noncontroversial part of the bidding and negotiation process. Medicare has been late to realize this concept, but Health Plan Employee Data and Information Set (HEDIS) 3.0 measures—a good place to start—are now required of all plans.

There are two types of objections to extensive data acquisition and dissemination requirements. First, consumers cannot properly interpret comparative quality measures, and therefore enrollees should receive only benefits information and the results of consumer satisfaction surveys. This could be called the FEHBP approach.

But even if not all buyers fully process the information, the provision of technical rankings and comparative performance data motivates sellers highly, since some buyers are fully informed and may act on the new information in the public domain. Examples include employer-sponsored health insurance markets (as reported by successful buyers), the market for air travel (as observed by passengers after on-time rankings became public), and automobile showrooms (each year when *Consumer Reports* publishes its issue on new cars). Medicare beneficiaries may turn to family members, peers, or their own support or advocacy groups to help them interpret and act on the comparative information. It is hard to imagine any beneficial effects on quality performance in a competitive insurance market without consumer information.

The second objection is that some plans are simply not organized to generate such data, and therefore they should not be held to the same reporting requirements as everyone else. This argument is often advanced by indemnity, PSO, PPO, and MSA advocates.

The implicit assumption here is that quality in these FFS-type arrangements is not at issue, and thus information collection and dissemination have no role to play. This assertion has been made in relation to FFS medicine ever since managed-care plans starting gaining market share. The clinical research literature suggests that the quality of care delivered in managed-care plans, on average, is no worse than that delivered in FFS settings and that quality everywhere could be substantially improved. The literature also clearly suggests that quality needs to be constantly monitored so that it can be improved by more effective dissemination of clinical best practices (President's Advisory Commission 1998), perhaps especially for Medicare enrollees. The decision not to demand data on quality from some plans and providers is an acceptance of the assertion. HCFA should not accept a mere assertion of impeccable FFS quality on behalf of Medicare beneficiaries.

**Step 4: Negotiate Competitive Bids with Plans.** There are two basic theories, each relied on to different degrees by different organized purchasers, of how competitive discipline is best imposed on health insurers: (1) through consumer reaction to price incentives and comparative quality information and (2) bilaterally through the sponsor negotiating directly with plans by using the combined monopsony power of the purchasing group. At the beginning of a new competitive bidding process, HCFA would be wise to try some of both. Some purchasers have found it useful to discuss plan-specific quality information quietly in lieu of public disclosure as a way of eliciting improved performance in the near future; some have also found it useful to threaten to deny access to their enrollees unless the first-round bid is lowered considerably. Organized purchasers report that they need about a 15 percent market share to exercise enough purchasing clout to get providers' attention and to demand accountability from their local health care systems. Medicare starts the game with enough clout in virtually every market in the country. There is no reason HCFA should not use this power.

**Step 5: Give Consumers Incentives to Choose Efficient Plans.** This is in some ways the most complicated and controversial step, because it entails setting the government contribution or contribution rule, that is, what the American people are willing to pay on behalf of Medicare+Choice enrollees. Given the distribution of bids and the risk-adjustment mechanism in place (step 6), this contribution rule determines the price incentives for beneficiaries. To facilitate the effect of incentives, plans should be allowed to offer rebates to enrollees if the government contribution exceeds their bid. Because current Medicare law does not permit plans to do this now, the plans essentially are forced to spend any savings on extra benefits.

Pure managed-competition theory calls for the sponsor—after ensuring that all participating plans are of acceptable quality and informing potential enrollees about what is known as to quality differences across plans—to set its premium contribution (a defined contribution, assuming beneficiaries will still pay their Part B premium, or $p$, to the program) at some fraction of the lowest bid for the standard benefit package and thus give the enrollee the maximum incentive to avoid high-cost plans. Though conceptually appealing and arguably the contribution rule most likely to retard the cost growth of premiums, this pure rule would present difficulties for Medicare to implement for three reasons.

First, low-cost plans might not have sufficient capacity to accommodate all Medicare beneficiaries who wish to join Medicare+Choice plans. The standard of low-cost plans could force some elderly to make extra out-of-pocket payments just to obtain coverage or could force them back into FFS Medicare. Second, tying the government contribution to the lowest bid raises the specter of a two-tiered Medicare program: low-income beneficiaries enrolling in low-cost plans and higher-income beneficiaries sorting themselves into more expensive plans. Without adequate quality monitoring, some advocates rightly worry about the long-term implications of two tiers.

The third argument against setting the government contribution at the bid of the lowest plan is the reality that many beneficiaries enjoy supplementary benefits at zero premium today. A pricing strategy for a low-cost plan would probably force most plans to charge a premium for supplemental benefits. This outcome would engender considerable beneficiary resistance, since the first result of competitive bidding would be a benefit reduction or an out-of-pocket cost increase. An alternative would be to define the standard benefit package as basic Medicare benefits plus the usual managed-care cost-sharing reduction, an out-of-pocket limit, and limited prescription drug coverage. The government contribution level could be set at the lowest-cost bid for these services, and then beneficiaries could sort themselves according to their wishes, given the incentives this would entail. The growth of costs over time is much more important to the ultimate social cost of the Medicare program than a one-time increase in benefit levels. Some local discretion could determine the benefits to which the government contribution would be pegged—for the same amount of money will surely go further in some places than in others.

Alternative rules for the government contribution offer trade-offs of incentive effects for equity and less pressure for omniscient (and immediate) quality monitoring of low-cost plans. There are two classes of useful rules: (1) a defined contribution set (arbitrarily) higher than the low-cost plan and (2) the government contribution set equal to a fixed percentage (say, 90 percent) of whatever plan the beneficiary picks. The percentage rule is likely to be less effective in curtailing cost growth, since the government shares in the extra expense of high-cost plans. I recommend the arbitrary defined-contribution rule, although no compelling logic sets it at any particular place in the distribution of bids.

The rule should be set according to local conditions. A benchmark might be the median bid for the benefit package that is defined as standard in a given area. If enrollment capacity in the plans that met some quality threshold and that bid at or below the median was more than adequate to accommodate most low-income Medicare beneficiaries in a given area, then the government could accomplish its objectives by setting the payment amount lower, for example, at the fortieth percentile bid. Conversely, if the combined capacity were inadequate for this purpose, one could raise the percentile of the bid distribution at which the defined contribution was set. The twin goals are to encourage plans to bid lower than the median and to ensure plan choice for lower-income Medicare beneficiaries. This delicate trade-off will likely evolve over time and will surely be handled best with local discretion by the HCFA bid manager.

**Step 6: Adjust Plan Payments by Risk**. Health plan competition must coexist with very skewed distribution of health expenditures: 10 percent of Medicare beneficiaries account for about 70 percent of Medi-

care spending in a given year (HCFA 1997). Plans at risk for beneficiary services have strong incentives to avoid beneficiaries who are more
likely to be high cost. To ensure that plan competition is focused on the
efficiency of delivery systems and the efficacy of the care delivered,
and not enrollee risk selection, premium payments to plans should reflect the relative risk of specific enrollees. Some, but surprisingly not
most, organized purchasers in the private and public sectors use a form
of risk adjustment. HCFA has spent considerable resources to research
the best risk adjuster for Medicare beneficiaries. A new system that is
approximately 50 percent more accurate than the current one is sched-
uled to be implemented on January 1, 2000.

Although it may be the best current system for Medicare, it is
hardly perfect. Three questions remain. Should required beneficiary
premium payments somewhat reflect their relative risks? Should plans
bid for a standard-risk enrollee only, or should they reveal their preferred ratios of payments for different risk classes; that is, should they
bid a matrix for each benefit package? Should a blended-risk adjuster,
part prospective, part retrospective, be used for at least the early years
of competitive bidding?

The first two questions are related. If the plan's internal expectations about relative risk factors differ from HCFA's calculations, then
HCFA's premium payments may encourage or discourage enrollment of
certain types of beneficiaries. For those for whom HCFA underpays (by
the plan's lights), the plan could be persuaded to take them willingly (and
not chase them away) if the beneficiary could be charged the difference.
This adjustment would enhance competition on the merits, but it would
require presumably higher-risk beneficiaries to pay more than lower-
risk beneficiaries for the same coverage. This arrangement comports
with the traditional insurance principle that higher-risk people pay an
amount correlated with their relative risk. But it violates the equity principle that considers health and risk status to be mostly random and
argues for personal payments to be uncorrelated with risk. Requiring
higher payments from higher-risk individuals deviates from traditional
Medicare philosophy. Still, perhaps one demonstration of competitive
bidding should consider experimenting with this in a limited way. The
benefits from the added competition and reduced risk segmentation
may be worthwhile, especially if higher premium payments could be
limited to higher-risk individuals who also have higher incomes.

The third question stems from long-standing recommendations by
Joseph Newhouse (Newhouse 1994; Newhouse, Buntin, and Chapman
1997), vice-chairman of Congress's Medicare Payment Advisory Com-

mission (MedPAC): since all prospective risk-adjustment systems are imperfect, Medicare should consider a weighted average between a purely prospective risk-adjustment payment and a retrospective component that could be triggered in an extremely high-cost case. While this blend would attenuate care-management incentives somewhat, it would also attenuate stinting incentives with a bad outcome, as well as reduce insurer efforts to avoid potential high-cost cases. Exploring this sensible correction for imperfect prospective risk adjustment would be worthwhile in at least one competitive bidding demonstration; reinsurance may also have an effect on the average and the distribution of premium bids.

## Conclusion

Would effective market competition of the type described in this chapter guarantee the 1 percent real rate of cost growth per beneficiary that so many Medicare reform plans assume? Probably not, for there are no guarantees in the real world. There is no magic solution to Medicare's financing problem. We are not likely to set in stone the precise structural rules that will or even should remain unchanged for thirty more years. There will be mistakes, adjustments, and productive evolution of perceived needs, rules, and benefits over time.

Any serious Medicare restructuring effort, as former senator Robert Dole pointed out (1997), will require sacrifice and change from all parts of the program and from all parts of society. The Part A trust fund shortfall must be addressed in the short run and probably entails some tax increases down the road in the longer run. But with competitive bidding, a defined benefit package, and accountable health plans, we could create the infrastructure that would facilitate collective decisions about exactly what we are willing to pay for, as promised medical value and current opportunity cost are weighed by the people's representatives in Congress.

Although we may end up with tax increases if we decide collectively that we want to pay for more health technology as it becomes available, we need not start there. We should start with a serious effort at restructuring Medicare along workable market lines, not ideologically pure free-market lines, but structured market lines. A competitive health plan market can be the Medicare program's best long-run friend, but only if we structure the relationship carefully. We can do so, and the time to start is this very momemt. We will all be Medicare beneficiaries soon enough.

# Notes

1. I simplify a bit by assuming there are no nonelderly disabled beneficiaries and no elderly workers, and that all public funds are financed with a payroll tax. Including the precise details would complicate the algebra without changing the essential point at all, since the general fund financing that reduces the actual required payroll tax rate also increases the fraction of income tax revenue that must be dedicated to Medicare. Nevertheless, the *t* that is calculated in this simplified example is higher than actually required because of current income tax financing and because of the payroll and income generated by elderly workers.

2. Author's calculations, details available on request.

# References

Butler, Stuart A., and Robert E. Moffit. 1995. "The FEHBP as a Model for a New Medicare Program." *Health Affairs* 14 (winter): 47–61.

Dole, Robert J. 1997. "Medicare: Let's Fix It." *Washington Post*, February 23.

Dowd, Bryan E., Roger Feldman, and Jon Christianson. 1996. *Competitive Pricing for Medicare.* Washington, D.C.: AEI Press.

Enthoven, Alain C., and Sara J. Singer. 1996. "Managed Competition and California's Health Care Economy." *Health Affairs* 15 (spring): 39–57.

Feldman, Roger, and Bryan E. Dowd. 1998. "Structuring Choice Under Medicare." In *Medicare: Preparing for the Challenges of the Twenty-first Century,* edited by Robert D. Reischauer, Stuart Butler, and Judith Lave. Washington, D.C.: National Academy of Social Insurance.

Jones, Stan. 1998. "The Medicare Beneficiary as Consumer." In *Medicare: Preparing for the Challenges of the Twenty-first Century,* edited by Robert D. Reischauer, Stuart Butler, and Judith Lave. Washington, D.C.: National Academy of Social Insurance.

Maxwell, James, Forrest Briscoe, Stephen Davidson, Lisa Eisen, Mark Robbins, Peter Temin, and Cheryl Young. 1998. "Managed Competition in Practice: 'Value Purchasing' by Fourteen Employers." *Health Affairs* 17 (May–June): 216–26.

Meyer, Jack A., Sharon Silow-Carroll, Ingrid A. Tillman, and Lise S. Rybowski. 1997. *Employer Coalition Initiatives in Health Care Purchasing.* Pt. 1, 2. Washington, D.C.: Economic and Social Research Institute.

Newhouse, Joseph P. 1994. "Patients at Risk: Health Reform and Risk Adjustment." *Health Affairs* 13 (spring): 132–46.

———. 1996. "Reimbursing Health Plans and Health Providers: Efficiency in Production versus Selection." *Journal of Economic Literature* 34 (September): 1236–63.

Newhouse, Joseph P., Melinda Beeuwkes Buntin, and John D. Chapman. 1997. "Risk Adjustment and Medicare: Taking a Closer Look." *Health Affairs* 16 (September–October): 26–43.

President's Advisory Commission on Quality in the Health Care Industry. 1998. *Quality First: Better Health Care for All Americans.* Washington, D.C.: Government Printing Office (http://www.hcqualitycommission.gov/final/).

Rice, Thomas, Marcia L. Graham, and Peter D. Fox. 1997. "The Impact of Policy Standardization on the Medigap Market." *Inquiry* 34 (summer): 106–16.

Robinson, James C., and Patricia E. Powers. 1998. "Restructuring Medicare: The Role of Public and Private Purchasing Alliances." In *Medicare: Preparing for the Challenges of the Twenty-first Century,* edited by Robert D. Reischauer, Stuart Butler, and Judith Lave. Washington, D.C.: National Academy of Social Insurance.

U.S. Health Care Financing Administration. 1997. *Health Care Financing Review: Medicare and Medicaid Statistical Supplement.* Washington, D.C.: Government Printing Office.

———. 1998. *A Profile of Medicare: Chart Book.* Washington, D.C.: Government Printing Office.

# 6

---

# The Forgotten Opportunity of Reforming Fee-for-Service Medicare

## H. E. Frech III

Medicare is a costly and rapidly growing program. At currently projected growth rates, it is the wild card in the debate over the political viability of Social Security. The all-important Medicare growth rate is hard to predict: forecasting the pension aspect of Social Security is child's play in comparison.

Even from the perspective of public choice, more than dollars is at stake. Medicare's efficiency is critical. An inefficient Medicare program, even if low-cost, would be a political problem (Bohn 1998) for Social Security: the extra burden on the program would reduce political support and viability. Conversely, even if costly, an efficient Medicare program would be highly valued by consumers and voters and would not be a political problem for Social Security.

Yet, discussion of Medicare reform is incomplete and even otherworldly.[1] It is dominated by the assumption that the future of Medicare is managed care. Although this may be true in the long run, as of

---

This essay is based on testimony before the Senate Budget Committee, delivered in 1997.

now managed care is only the tail, not the dog. The dog is traditional fee-for-service Medicare. More than 80 percent of Medicare beneficiaries are still in fee-for-service plans. Inefficiencies in traditional Medicare, discussed below, are doubly wasteful. They make traditional Medicare artificially attractive and thus slow the shift into managed care.

On the rare occasions when traditional Medicare is actually discussed, the issues are typically minor changes in payments (for example, further reducing the payments made to hospitals and physicians, changing the accounting for home health care). These complex discussions are rewarding only for those with immediate budgetary responsibility and those representing special interests such as teaching hospitals, physicians, or home health care companies.

Surprisingly, the most promising place to begin thinking about reform is traditional Medicare, which presents great room for improvement. For historical and political reasons, traditional Medicare was poorly designed. Congress did build in cost controls, in the form of consumer cost-sharing for hospital care and especially for physician care. But the growth of private supplementary Medigap coverage has almost completely destroyed these cost controls.[2] Even partially reversing this process would provide major improvements. Costs could be decreased while efficiency would be improved.

What is more, the movement of Medicare beneficiaries into managed care has been slowed by the existence of Medigap. Eliminating or discouraging Medigap would remove this artificial barrier to the growth of managed care and lead to further long-run efficiency gains.

## The Long-Run Movement into Managed Care

Despite the subsidies to traditional Medicare, substantial numbers of Medicare beneficiaries have substantially moved into managed care. Between 1990 and 1995, the percentage of beneficiaries enrolled in Medicare health maintenance organizations (HMOs) grew from 3.3 to 8.8 percent (MedPAC 1998, 4–5).[3]

Growth in Medicare HMOs trails the growth of managed care in the private sector. By 1995, even by conservative definitions, 72 percent of Americans with insurance were in managed-care plans: 26 percent in HMOs, 5 percent in the point-of-service (POS) plans, and 41 percent in preferred-provider (PPO) plans.[4] Both POSs and PPOs are more flexible than traditional HMOs. They allow the consumer to go outside the network to receive care from nonmember providers and still retain some insurance coverage. These plans have grown much faster than HMOs.

It is useful to take a wider view of managed care, including plans with utilization management (for example, precertification of admission, utilization review). With managed care defined this way, the percentages of nonelderly Americans with managed care are still higher. According to a 1991 Health Insurance Institute of America survey of employer-provided insurance, conventional insurance with utilization management covered 38 percent of employees, while conventional insurance without utilization management covered a mere 8 percent (Sullivan, Miller, Feldman, and Dowd 1992, 176). As early as 1991, truly unmanaged insurance had all but disappeared from the private sector.

If we adjust the more recent surveys by the percentage with utilization management, managed care for the nonelderly is even more dominant.[5] By 1995, 95 percent of working-age insured Americans were in some category of managed-care plans (26 percent in HMOs, 5 percent in POS plans, 41 percent in PPO plans, and 23 percent in utilization-management-only plans). Traditional HMOs, the only managed-care option of any importance in Medicare, account for only about one-fourth of managed-care enrollments. The vast majority are in much more flexible managed-care systems.

In the long run, most Medicare beneficiaries probably will choose managed care of one kind or another, just as most working-age consumers have. This will be beneficial to cost-control and efficiency.[6] For both unavoidable market reasons and avoidable policy reasons, this shift will be much slower than for working-age consumers. Medicare's traditional fee-for-service coverage will remain important for a long time. As long as drastic and punitive regulations or price controls are not imposed on fee-for-service medicine, managed care will not dominate for perhaps thirty years. Even in the medium term, Medicare fee-for-service insurance cannot be ignored.

## Medicare Fee-for-Service and Cost-Sharing

**Fee-for-Service Medicare Is Inefficient.** Medicare's benefit structure was essentially copied from Blue Cross/Blue Shield plans of the early 1960s. Although it was not obvious in 1965, Medicare began with an inefficient benefit design. It is sometimes said that Medicare has a 1965 state-of-the-art benefit structure. Even this faint praise is too much.

Medicare's benefit structure was not even state-of-the-art for 1965. Because it was based on Blue Cross/Blue Shield, it inherited several traditional Blue Cross/Blue Shield features that are now generally regarded as mistakes.

First, Blue Cross/Blue Shield insurance was overly complete. It had substantially less cost-sharing (deductibles, coinsurance, and balance-billing) than commercial insurers. This was natural since the Blues were founded and originally controlled by hospitals and physicians, who had an obvious incentive for more complete insurance. Further, promoting relatively complete coverage was a purposeful part of Blue Cross/Blue Shield philosophy, expressed in the national requirements for approval and the use of the Blue Cross and Blue Shield trademarks (Frech 1996, 108–11). The overly complete nature of Blue Cross/Blue Shield coverage exacerbated the subsidy or moral hazard problem of health insurance and raised demand, utilization, and prices more than necessary. Even as early as 1969, areas with high Blue Cross/Blue Shield market shares had higher hospital costs, utilization, and prices than areas where the Blue plans were less important (Frech 1979; Frech and Ginsburg 1978; Hay and Leahy 1984).[7]

Second, Medicare does not cover many important medical costs. Again, following the structure of the Blue Cross/Blue Shield of the 1960s, Medicare focuses on inpatient hospital and physician costs. This structure causes Medicare beneficiaries to be exposed to substantial financial risk, even if they are not terribly sick, if they do not have private Medigap or Medicaid coverage of those other services. Commercial insurance was already rectifying this problem as early as the 1960s by covering a wide variety of services with a major medical component.

Third, Medicare's benefit structure is upside-down from the viewpoint of efficient insurance. It covers the first dollars of hospital and physician care relatively completely, but its coverage of catastrophic events is poor. The most glaring example is inpatient hospital coverage. After a deductible, the first 60 days of hospitalization are 100 percent covered. But then the beneficiary pays $191 per day for days 61–90 and $382 per day for days 91–150. After day 150, hospital inpatient bills are not covered at all. While this shallow coverage was common in early Blue Cross, it contrasts sharply with modern private insurance, which usually has stop-loss amounts, beyond which the consumer pays nothing. By 1993, more than 80 percent of employees in non-HMOs had stop-losses. These stop-loss limits are generally fairly low, with an average of $1,319 for large and medium-size private firms (EBRI 1995, 312–13). A Medicare-only beneficiary can easily go far beyond that level.

The structure of Medicare benefits does an amazingly poor job of risk-spreading. It exposes beneficiaries to substantial financial risk because of uncovered services and because of poor coverage of catastrophic events. Data from the 1987 National Medical Expenditures Survey (NMES) show that a Medicare-only beneficiary at the seventy-fifth percentile in total spending would be responsible for $2,591 in cost-sharing and direct payment for services. A beneficiary at the ninetieth percentile would be responsible for $9,472 (Miller 1998). This situation induces more beneficiaries to purchase Medigap insurance to reduce their exposure to financial risk.

**Private Supplemental (Medigap) Coverage Is Destructive.** The only cost-control mechanism in Medicare fee-for-service insurance is its cost-sharing. Private supplementary insurance (employer group supplements and individually purchased Medigap) has largely destroyed the cost control built into Medicare by filling in deductibles and coinsurance and, in some cases, even paying balance bills.[8]

Over the years, supplemental insurance has been allowed to grow from only 46 percent in 1967 (Taylor, Short, and Horgan 1988, 149) to about 72 percent of Medicare beneficiaries in 1995. An additional number (about 15 percent) have Medicaid coverage that also fills in the cost-sharing. This supplemental insurance reduces or undermines Medicare's cost-control (PPRC 1997, 318–19). Medicare's original cost control system is intact only for the 13 percent of consumers who have neither Medigap nor Medicaid coverage. This is the single most serious problem with the program.

Beneficiaries with supplemental insurance consume much more care, which greatly raises the cost to Medicare. Most of this extra spending becomes an extra burden to Medicare. Economists have studied this effect extensively (see Christensen and Shingole 1997; Chulis et al. 1993; Taylor, Short and Horgan 1988). Recently, the Physician Payment Review Commission (PPRC) has estimated that Medicare beneficiaries with private supplemental insurance consume 28 percent more care than those with Medicare only.[9] Medicare pays for most of the extra utilization costs, about $1,000 extra per beneficiary (PPRC 1996, 291, 292). The total extra cost imposed on Medicare by Medigap insurance is about 20 percent of the total Medicare budget, or about $30 billion.

This shifting of the burden to Medicare is what economists call an *externality*. Through this externality, Medicare provides a large subsidy for insurance that undermines Medicare's own cost controls. Further, employee group supplemental coverage also benefits from the general tax subsidy of health insurance. Employees are not taxed for the economic benefit of health insurance, yet employers can deduct the premiums as a regular cost of doing business. In two ways, then, the government subsidizes supplemental insurance that is destructive of its own budgetary goal of controlling cost, as well as being destructive of economic efficiency.

Beyond ruining Medicare's cost controls, as discussed below, supplementary insurance artificially slows progress toward more use of managed care. And the distributional effects of allowing Medigap insurance are perverse. On average, consumers with supplementary coverage are wealthier than those without it.

**The Poor Elderly and Medicare/Medicaid Crossovers.** The poor elderly can be, and generally are, covered by both Medicaid and Medicare. For almost all of these dually eligible (also called *crossover*) beneficiaries, Medicaid pays the premium for Part B (physician services insurance) and fills in the cost-sharing and covers other services (PPRC 1997, 6–7). The combination of programs amounts to comprehensive insurance coverage indeed. In 1997, the average Medicare-only beneficiary paid $1,273 per year in cost-sharing. In contrast, the average dually eligible beneficiary paid only $265 per year in cost-sharing (AARP 1997, 7, 13).

In effect, the combination of the programs provides income-related cost-sharing, a policy that has been suggested by health economists for many years.[10] The elderly with low-enough income to qualify for Medicaid along with Medicare have extremely complete insurance coverage. A recent study by Katie Merrell, David Colby, and Christopher Hogan showed that 73.9 percent of the dually eligible beneficiaries had income below $10,000 in 1993. The figure for those without Medicaid coverage was only 24.9 (1997, 178). The crossover program is generally a sensible policy.[11] This Medicaid/Medicare policy allows Congress to reform Medicare efficiently and appropriately for the majority of the elderly who are not poor, without concern that higher cost-sharing might sometime be a major problem for low-income elderly.

# Suggested Reforms in Fee-for-Service Medicare

**Prohibit or Discourage Supplemental Insurance.** The most important immediate reform of Medicare would be to prohibit or discourage Medigap policies that fill in Medicare's cost-sharing.[12] The savings that could be achieved by reinstating even part of the original cost controls are great. This could be done many ways, including simple prohibition, a tax reflecting the harm done to Medicare by Medigap supplements, integration of Medigap with Medicare, and reform of Medicare benefits to discourage Medigap supplements. Not mutually exclusive, these policies could be combined.

The prohibition of Medigap coverage sounds authoritarian and radical. Yet it represents a smaller change in policy than one might think. Since 1992, Congress has intervened heavily in the individual Medigap market (about half of Medigap is individual and half group). Certain types of coverage have, in fact, been prohibited, while others have been required: only ten types of individual Medigap policies can be sold (Rice, Graham, and Fox 1997). Unfortunately, the individual Medigap regulation has been so poorly designed that coverage of Part B physician coinsurance is actually required, rather than prohibited!

There are three major cost controls: Part B coinsurance, Part B deductibles, and Part A hospital deductibles. Unfortunately for cost control, the regulation of Medigap plans has resulted in sales of Part B deductible insurance more than doubling, from 21–27 percent to 58 percent (Rice, Graham, and Fox 1997, 111).

One could take the same administrative approach and simply prohibit all Medigap plans that negate the three important cost controls mentioned above. Although it would be administratively more difficult, Congress could extend the provisions to employer-provided group Medigap coverage.

Health economists (for example, Paul Ginsburg 1982, 54–55) have proposed taxing Medigap policies. Such a policy reflects the economics of harmful externalities. Assume that all Medigap policies can be represented by the average policy. PPRC research has estimated that the average Medigap policy raises Medicare costs by about $1,000 per beneficiary. Therefore, $1,000 is an estimate of the harm imposed on Medicare when the average consumer buys the average Medigap policy. The ideal tax on an externality is equal to the harm caused by that externality: the appropriate tax on Medigap policies would be about $1,000.

Since the average premium for Medigap policies was about $1,014 in 1992, this tax would roughly double the cost of Medigap insurance (PPRC 1996, 282–83). Earlier, using 1977 data, I had calculated a somewhat larger tax rate of 124 percent (Frech 1988, 11–13).

Tax solutions for such externality problems have characteristic vices and virtues. A major virtue is transparency. The source, direction, and magnitude of the externality are clear in the tax itself. Conversely, the tax solution is crude. In reality, there are many types of Medigap insurance, with different effects on cost control and thus with different amounts of external harm done to Medicare. (For example, despite recent increases, about 40 percent of Medigap does not cover the Part B deductible).[13] Further, there are regional and demographic differences in the magnitude of the effect. An efficient tax system should take account of at least some of these differences.

An alternative approach is integrating Medigap and Medicare. This plan would require that the Medigap insurer become responsible for paying all costs of Medicare. The PPRC (1996, 301–3) and the Congressional Budget Office (1991) have suggested that the Medigap insurer be required to cover all Medicare-covered services itself. In return for shouldering the entire burden, Medicare would pay the integrated firm a fixed capitated amount, much as it currently does for HMOs. As with HMOs, such capitation requires complex risk-adjusting for the Medicare payment or tolerating some overpayment and thus raises the possibility of inefficient risk-sorting. But the possible gains, as shown above, are enormous.

This system of integrated insurance would accomplish the same end as the tax solution and would be in some ways worse and in some ways better. Integrated insurance would not be so transparent. Consumers and outsiders would observe only the price of Medigap insurance. They could not see how much of that price was accounted for by the external harms to Medicare, in contrast to the intrinsic cost of the insurance. Conversely, integration would automatically pick up the differences in the external effects. All extra cost imposed on Medicare would be internalized (paid by the Medigap insurer). An inefficient benefit structure with major effects on demand and costs would impose high costs on the insurer. A more moderate system would impose lower costs.

The American Medical Association has suggested a different approach (1997, 13–16). The AMA suggested modernizing Medicare benefits by making them more like modern fee-for-service insurance. The new Medicare would cover all or most services, including the hospital costs associated with catastrophic events, and would carry a uniform deductible. This reform would make Medigap insurance less attractive, so that relatively few beneficiaries (or their employers) would purchase it. As discussed above, an important reason for beneficiaries to purchase Medigap policies is the large remaining financial risk caused by Medicare's poorly designed benefit structure. If the inherent financial risk of Medicare alone were dramatically reduced, the demand for Medigap policies would decline.

The exact cost-saving of this plan would depend on beneficiaries' demand responses. Some beneficiaries might still demand Medigap insurance, again with the large harmful externality discussed above. This outcome seems especially likely for those with employer-provided Medigap coverage. While reduced, the external harm to Medicare would still exist and might continue to induce consumers to purchase Medigap coverage and employers to provide Medigap coverage for their retirees.[14] Although the AMA does not mention it, this approach could easily be combined with a prohibition of, or tax on, any remaining Medigap insurance or with integration.

Indeed, any reasonably modern reform of Medicare's benefit structure would adopt, more or less, the AMA's suggested form (coverage of more services; deeper, or right-side-up, coverage; coordinated deductibles; stop-loss levels). And, intended or not, the reform would make Medigap coverage less attractive and less common.

**Introduce Options for Expanded Cost-Sharing.** At the same time, options for expanded cost-sharing, most likely in the form of a large-deductible catastrophic policy, should be introduced. This could be done simply and directly. But the direct approach may not be politically acceptable because of the inability of the government to commit to holding beneficiaries to their high cost-sharing plan if they become poor.

Consider this scenario. Some Medicare beneficiaries with mid- to high-income and asset levels would choose high cost-sharing plans. Later, for some of these beneficiaries, assets and incomes would fall, perhaps because of high levels of nonmedical spending or risky investments. Therefore, these insureds would become low-income beneficiaries; the high cost-sharing plan could lead to financial hardship and low consumption of medical care. This outcome might be politically unacceptable. The government would be likely to bail them out, as it already does low-income Medicare beneficiaries through Medicaid coverage. The expectation that the government would bail out the unlucky beneficiaries encourages the irresponsible risk-taking behavior in the first place.

This problem could be avoided by requiring those who choose high cost-sharing plans to maintain some savings to pay the cost-sharing amount. One possibility receiving attention in the United States and Singapore is the concept of a medical savings account. Another possibility is structuring deductibles as rebates or refunds of premiums for good experience, as is common in German health insurance (Zweifel 1988, 1992).

## Medicare Managed Care

**Unavoidable market reasons.** Movement into managed care will be slow for Medicare beneficiaries. Managed care is less attractive to the elderly than to younger consumers. (One can see the same forces at work in the greater acceptance of managed care by the young within the work force.) The elderly are more likely to have developed personal relationships with one or more physicians. They want to maintain this relationship when they retire and are generally resistant to managed care, especially to the traditional HMO, which pays zero benefits for out-of-plan care. This is not mere sentimentality or inertia. Continuing, long-term patient-physician relationships have important medical benefits. As a result, movement into managed care will be slower for the elderly than for working-age consumers.

The private market has developed a range of managed-care options, from utilization-control-only plans to traditional HMOs with small, closed physician panels.[15] Even for working-age consumers, the relatively flexible plans have strongly outperformed the traditional HMOs. For the elderly, the forces leading to better performance by more-flexible managed-care plans are even stronger.

**Avoidable Policy Reasons.** Medicare policy has slowed movement of beneficiaries into more-efficient managed-care systems. First, Medicare's permissive approach to, and the tax subsidy of, Medigap insurance have made Medicare fee-for-service artificially attractive. With supplementary insurance, many beneficiaries have approximately 100 percent coverage, without the utilization-control or provider-choice limits of managed care. In fact, Medicare with Medigap coverage is virtually the only place where 100 percent, first-dollar coverage still exists.

Further, the existing Medicare managed-care option is the least attractive and beneficial type for the elderly. The most attractive type of managed care for the elderly is a more flexible plan that would provide some benefits for continuing to see out-of-plan physicians. That is, the more-flexible managed-care plans, such as PPOs and POS plans, are likely to be the most attractive and most beneficial for the elderly. Yet only restrictive, traditional HMOs have been offered them on any scale.

This problem has been recognized recently. In 1995, the Health Care Financing Administration announced that a POS option could be offered to Medicare HMO beneficiaries. By 1997, this option was available to about 10 percent of those with Medicare HMO coverage (PPRC 1997, 23). A recent change in law will ultimately broaden the choice of managed-care plans. The Medicare+Choice feature of the Balanced Budget Act of 1997 is intended to allow a larger array of managed-care plans to compete for Medicare beneficiaries (PPRC 1997, 4–5).

## Conclusion

Managed care has many advantages, including lower costs. But the option has so captured the attention of analysts and policymakers that the opportunity for reform of traditional Medicare has been overlooked. Traditional Medicare fee-for-service is dominant. Movement into Medicare HMOs has been, and will continue to be, slow.

The spectacular growth of Medigap insurance has undermined the basic cost-controls built into Medicare at its founding. Medigap imposes major external harm on Medicare: an extra burden of about 20 percent of Medicare expenditures, or about $30 billion per year. Discouraging Medigap coverage could reap huge savings. This reform would also encourage movement into Medicare managed care. Modernizing the antique and inefficient Medicare benefit structure also offers important gains. In an unusual two for one, modernizing Medicare benefits would, by itself, discourage harmful Medigap coverage.

## Notes

1. A recent study that supposedly focused on fee-for-service Medicare decided explicitly not to address increasing beneficiary cost-sharing or changing the fee-for-service benefit structure. The study analyzed only the addition of managed-care features to traditional Medicare (NASI 1998). In other words,

the study group ruled out basic reforms of traditional fee-for-service Medicare from the start.

2. The term *Medigap* is sometimes reserved for individually purchased private supplementary coverage. I use the word in the more general sense to include all private supplementary coverage, including that provided by current or previous employers.

3. This refers to Medicare-risk HMOs only. Medicare-cost HMOs, despite the name, function as ordinary fee-for-service providers.

4. While still greatly lagging behind the private market, the Medicare percentage in HMOs grew to 14.0 percent by 1997.

5. The adjustment requires multiplying the percentage with fee-for-service coverage by the ratio of fee-for-service with utilization management to fee-for-service with no utilization management: (28 percent)(38 percent/46 percent) = 23 percent.

6. Sandra Christensen and Judy Shinogle find impressive cost reductions from Medicare HMOs. They (1997, 12) estimate that Medicare HMO beneficiaries use about 4 percent less total services than the next lowest group, Medicare-only beneficiaries.

7. Recent research suggests that this historic relationship has weakened and perhaps disappeared as the Blue plans have lost market power and have been forced to be more competitive. Stephen Foreman, John Anderson Wilson, and Richard Scheffler (1996) have shown the high Blue Cross market share is related to lower Blue Cross costs in more recent years.

8. Balance bills arise when the insurer's allowed payment is less than the total bill. The consumer is then billed for the balance. Once quite common, balance billing is still an important aspect of consumer cost-sharing in Medicare. See Frech 1996, 13, 14. As an example, on January 17, 1997, *CNN Headline News* ran a commercial for a Physician's Mutual Insurance supplemental policy specifically touting it for filling in the deductible and coinsurance and even for paying balance bills.

9. This estimate of 28 percent higher spending is about what one would expect. The classic RAND Health Insurance Experiment found expenses about 18–23 percent higher with free care than with 25 percent coinsurance (Newhouse 1993, 40–45).

10. For early examples, see Feldstein 1971 and Pauly 1979.

11. While the basic features of the Medicaid/Medicare crossover program make sense, there may be efficiency problems with this group. A warning flag is the fact that the dually eligible population consumes a large amount of medical care, more than twice as much in Medicare-covered services as those with Medicare only and about 65 percent more than those with private Medigap

coverage (PPRC 1996, 291; Merrell, Colby, and Horgan 1997, 179). Further, this small population consumes about 70 percent of total Medicaid spending (CBO 1997, 39). Still, the high spending is not entirely due to different incentives, since the dually eligible population is, on average, in poorer health than other populations.

12. It seems most likely that supplementary policies that cover other services, but do not fill in the cost-sharing, do not need to be prohibited, or discouraged. Examples would include paying for hospitalization beyond Medicare's limits and outpatient drug coverage. However, these policies might create incentive problems, especially if the coverage is overly complete for small losses. Further research on this issue would be welcome.

13. Christensen and Shinogle (1997, 12) find a larger demand-increasing effect from individual Medigap polices than from group polices. The individual policies typically have less cost-sharing than the group policies.

14. As Mark Pauly has shown (1974), the externality imposed by supplemental insurance on a primary insurance system always provides an extra incentive to overinsurance. This is an inherent problem in allowing supplemental insurance to be sold by separate, unintegrated, and untaxed insurers. The problem is reduced but not completely eliminated by Medicare benefit reform to reduce financial risk and to discourage Medigap.

15. Most of the more flexible plans, especially PPOs, benefit from combining cost-sharing with managed-care utilization controls. For historical and philosophical reasons, HMOs have resisted cost-sharing. But there is no logical or theoretical reason why cost-sharing and managed care should be considered mutually exclusive. Many efficient plans will probably combine both methods of cost control.

# References

American Association of Retired Persons, Public Policy Institute and the Lewin Group. 1997. *Out-of-Pocket Health Spending by Medicare Beneficiaries Age 65 and Older: 1997 Projections.* Washington, D.C.: AARP.

American Medical Association. 1997. *Transforming Medicare.* Chicago: AMA.

Bohn, Henning. 1998. "Will Social Security and Medicare Remain Viable As the U.S. Is Aging?" Working Paper 5-98. University of California, Santa Barbara, Department of Economics.

Christensen, Sandra, and Judy Shinogle. 1997. "Effects of Supplemental Coverage on Use of Services by Medicare Enrollees." *Health Care Financing Review* 19 (1) (fall): 5–17.

Chulis, George S., Franklin J. Eppig, Mary O. Hogan, Daniel R. Waldo, and Ross H. Arnet III. 1993. "Health Insurance and the Elderly: Data from the MCBS." *Health Care Financing Review* 14 (3) (spring): 163–81.

Congressional Budget Office. 1991. *Restructuring Health Insurance for Medical Enrollees.* Washington, D.C.: Government Printing Office.

————. 1997. *Long-Term Budgetary Pressures and Policy Options.* Washington, D.C.: Government Printing Office.

Employee Benefits Research Institute. 1995. *EBRI Databook on Employee Benefits.* Washington, D.C.: EBRI.

Feldstein, Martin S. 1971. "A New Approach to National Health Insurance." *Public Interest* (no. 23) (spring): 251–80.

Foreman, Stephen Earl, John Anderson Wilson, and Richard M. Scheffler. 1996. "Monopoly, Monopsony and Contestability in Health Insurance: A Study of Blue Cross Plans." *Economic Inquiry* 34 (4) (October): 662–77.

Frech, H. E. III. 1979. "Market Power in Health Insurance: Effects on Insurance and Medical Markets." *Journal of Industry Economics* 27 (1) (September): 55–72.

————. 1988. "Introduction." In *Health Care in America: The Political Economy of Hospitals and Health Insurance*, edited by H. E. Frech III. San Francisco: Pacific Research Institute for Public Policy.

————. 1996. *Competition and Monopoly in Medical Care.* Washington, D.C.: AEI Press.

Frech, H. E. III, and Paul B. Ginsburg. 1978. "Competition among Health Insurers." In *Competition in the Health Care Sector: Past, Present and Future*, edited by Warren Greenburg. Germantown, Md.: Aspen.

Ginsburg, Paul B. 1982. *Containing Medical Care Costs through Market Forces.* Washington, D.C.: Government Printing Office.

Hay, Joel W., and Michael J. Leahy. 1984. "Competition among Health Plans: Some Preliminary Evidence." *Southern Economic Journal* 50 (3) (January): 831–46.

Medicare Payment Advisory Commission. 1998. *Report to the Congress: Medicare Payment Policy.* Washington, D.C.: MedPAC.

Merrell, Katie, David C. Colby, and Christopher Hogan. 1997. "Medicare Beneficiaries Covered by Medicaid Buy-In Agreements." *Health Affairs* 16 (1) (January–February): 175–84.

Miller, Richard D. Jr. 1998. Private communication. May 11.

National Academy of Social Insurance. 1998. *From a Generation Behind to a Generation Ahead: Transforming Traditional Medicare.* Final report of the Study Panel on Fee-for-Service Medicare. Washington, D.C.: NASI.

Newhouse, Joseph P. 1993. *Free for All: Lessons from the RAND Health Insurance Experiment.* Cambridge, Mass.: Insurance Experiment Group.

Pauly, Mark V. 1974. "Overinsurance and Public Provision of Insurance: The Roles of Moral Hazard and Adverse Selection." *Quarterly Journal of Economics* 88 (1) (February): 44–62.

————. 1979. *The Role of the Private Sector in National Health Insurance.* Washington, D.C.: Health Insurance Institute.

Physician Payment Review Commission. 1996. *Annual Report to Congress 1996.* Washington, D.C.: PPRC.

————. 1997. *Annual Report to Congress 1997.* Washington, D.C.: PPRC.

Rice, Thomas, Marcia L. Graham, and Peter D. Fox. 1997. "The Impact of Policy Standardization on the Medigap Market." *Inquiry* 34 (2) (summer): 106–16.

Sullivan, Cynthia B., Marianne Miller, Roger Feldman, and Bryan Dowd. 1992. "Employer-Sponsored Health Insurance in 1991." *Health Affairs* 11 (4) (winter): 172–84.

Taylor, Amy K., Pamela Farley Short, and Constance M. Horgan. 1988. "Medigap Insurance: Friend or Foe in Reducing Medicare Deficits?" In *Health Care in America: The Political Economy of Hospitals and Health Insurance,* edited by H. E. Frech III. San Francisco: Pacific Research Institute for Public Policy.

Zweifel, Peter. 1988. "Rebates for No Claims as a Copayment Scheme: The Experience of German Private Health Insurance." In *Health Care in America: The Political Economy of Hospitals and Health Insurance,* edited by H. E. Frech III. San Francisco: Pacific Research Institute for Public Policy.

————. 1992. *Bonus Options in Health Insurance.* Dordrecht: Kluwer.

# 7

# Issues in Competitive Pricing

## Bryan Dowd and Roger Feldman

The Medicare program continues to occupy center stage on the U.S. political agenda. The National Bipartisan Commission on Medicare met to address the fiscal problems faced by the program and to make recommendations for reform. The Competitive Pricing Advisory Commission, established under the Balanced Budget Act of 1997, has designed and chosen sites for a competitive-pricing demonstration project. In the context of this churning political environment, it is important not only to maintain perspective on the nature and extent of the problem but also to continue to think about the details of particular proposals and their long-run impact on the health insurance and health care delivery system for the elderly.

### Efficiency and Fairness Concerns about Medicare

Although most current discussion of Medicare focuses on fiscal solvency, particularly of Part A, our interest in Medicare reform has a dif-

The authors wish to acknowledge support by the Health Care Financing Administration. The views expressed in this chapter are those of the authors, and all mistakes are their responsibility.

124

ferent basis. We are concerned about the efficiency of the program, and our concerns would remain even if the program were on a sound financial footing. Viewed purely from a perspective of efficiency, looming insolvency merely makes pursuit of a desirable objective politically expedient.

While insolvency concerns do not drive our interest in increased program efficiency, the insolvency problem is integral to our concerns about the program's fairness. In reviewing the current Medicare program, McClellan and Skinner (1997) find that the program leads to "net transfers from the poor to the wealthy, as a result of relatively regressive financing mechanisms and the higher expenditures and longer survival times of wealthier beneficiaries."

Their analysis assumes that the Medicare program continues. But the threat of fiscal insolvency is the primary fairness problem associated with Medicare (Dowd and Feldman 1998). Medicare financing relies on a massive infusion of tax dollars from current workers who, under the present schedule of revenue and expenditures, have no legitimate hope of ever qualifying as beneficiaries. Changing that situation will involve a significant increase in new tax revenue or significant restructuring of the current program

If nothing is done to restrain Medicare expenditures, the Medicare trustees have estimated that the taxes on future generations needed to restore the program to fiscal solvency would increase from 3.4 percent of workers' earnings in 1997 to 7.8 percent in 2070 (Board of Trustees, HI 1998; Board of Trustees, SMI 1998).[1] The Medicare payroll tax is projected to rise from 3.16 percent to 10.11 percent of the wage base (Board of Trustees, HI 1995; Board of Trustees, SMI 1995). The political process will decide whether these tax rates are politically feasible. In any case, we concur with the Medicare trustees' suggestion that Congress "take additional actions to control HI program costs" (Board of Trustees, HI 1995, 28).

## Fair Approaches to Reducing Medicare Expenditures

We have earlier analyzed the fairness of different approaches to reduce Medicare expenditures (that issue, in turn, addresses the problem of intergenerational fairness) (Feldman and Dowd 1998). We concluded that across-the-board cuts in Medicare benefits are regressive, because they fall equally on all beneficiaries, regardless of their income.[2] Coverage of fewer services or increased point-of-purchase cost-sharing, for example, can be criticized on the grounds that the poor are less able to bear the additional cost than the wealthy.[3]

A second cost-cutting option is means-testing. Medicare is often portrayed as a social insurance program, but close inspection suggests that "insurance" is a misnomer. Insurance policies are written to cover the losses associated with risky events; a policy pays off only if the insured event occurs. If the purpose of the Medicare program is to ensure that all aged and disabled individuals and end-stage renal disease (ESRD) patients have health insurance, whether they can afford it or not, then the insured event seems to be the "attainment of program eligibility (by becoming aged, disabled or having ESRD) and being poor." In that context, oddly, the program "pays off" (provides benefits) even if the unfortunate event (eligibility plus poverty) does not occur.

A third approach to cost-cutting is merit-testing. Current Medicare beneficiaries represent a generation of people who, in their early twenties, fought a world war on two fronts and saved the Western world from unimaginable horror. They went on to build the strongest economy in history, protect civilization from nuclear annihilation, and run the Soviet Union, our largest, most oppressive, and most ambitious economic and political competitor, out of business. The children and the grandchildren of that generation may decide that those accomplishments more than merit the Medicare program's current, unsustainable income transfer—but only for that generation. Explicitly acknowledging that transfer, for that reason, would accomplish two things. First, stating the younger generation's gratitude with sufficient clarity might help correct the misconception of current beneficiaries that they are "paying their own way." Second, such a statement would allow us to begin discussions about appropriate financing for the next generation, which, because of sheer numbers, poses the greatest fiscal threat to the program—and to whom no such debt is owed.

A fourth approach to cost-cutting is limiting the government's contribution to Medicare premiums. Central to this discussion is the view of the Medicare entitlement as a defined benefit or a defined contribution. (That issue is the focus of the first part of this chapter.)

A final approach to cost-cutting is achieving greater efficiency in the cost of caring for beneficiaries and structuring the program so that the use of more efficient care actually reduces the program's costs. For the sake of this discussion, we define *greater efficiency* as achieving the same health outcome at lower cost. We assume that health plans vary in the degree to which they can achieve these efficiency gains, but they also vary in other ways that are of value to beneficiaries.

In the current Medicare program the relationship between the health plan chosen by the beneficiary and the cost to the program is tenuous, at best. When a beneficiary joined a health maintenance organization (HMO) under the payment system of adjusted average per capita costs (AAPCC), the program's costs were reduced, at most, 5 percent. Studies have indicated that the 5 percent savings were more than offset by favorable selection into HMOs (Brown et al. 1993).[4] The choice of a specific private health plan does not affect program costs because the government's contribution to premiums is not tied to health plan costs.

Under our proposal for competitive pricing (Dowd, Feldman, and Christianson 1996), the government's contribution to premiums is set at the price submitted by the lowest-priced qualified health plan in each market area.[5] Competitive pressure links the health plans' prices to their costs, and the low-bid contribution system links the health plans' costs to Medicare's costs. Under our system, Medicare's cost would fall immediately to the premium of the lowest-cost qualified health plan in the market area (minus the Part B premium paid by the beneficiary) for every beneficiary in the market area.

Previously (Dowd and Feldman 1998), we suggested that this withdrawal of the beneficiary's entitlement to fee-for-service (FFS) care for only the Part B premium was the fairest approach to reducing program benefits. That suggestion is based on several observations:

1. Managed-care plans with limited provider panels already are an integral part of the Medicare program. The 1997 Balanced Budget Act expanded the variety of private health plans that may contract with Medicare.

2. Most of the population younger than sixty-five are enrolled in some type of managed-care plan.

3. Anecdotes to the contrary, careful studies based on chart reviews and on data from National Cancer Institute's cancer registry (the Surveillance, Epidemiology, and End-Results Program, SEER) suggest that the quality of care for serious medical conditions in Medicare HMOs either equals or exceeds quality in the FFS sector (Carlisle et al. 1994; Retchin, Clement, and Brown 1994; Riley et al. 1994).

4. The demand for FFS plans in employment-based insurance relates positively to the employee's income (Cutler and Reber 1998), and thus the differential public subsidy of FFS delivery systems is regressive.

Competitive pricing for Medicare not only is a fair way to reduce government spending but also will result in a more efficient allocation of resources in two ways. First, better-informed beneficiaries will face the marginal cost of choosing more expensive health plans, after adjusting for enrollee risk-differentials; this situation will lead to a more efficient allocation of beneficiaries across plans. Second, the government will face a price of Medicare benefits that reflects costs in the most-efficient health plan in each market area, rather than costs in the FFS sector. As a result, the government can purchase a more efficient level of the Medicare entitlement.

The following sections explore issues central to the fourth and fifth approaches to reducing Medicare's costs. The first section discusses the Medicare entitlement as a defined-benefit, in contrast to a defined-contribution, program. The second section discusses problems with achieving the optimally efficient distribution of enrollees across health plans offered in the market area.

## Defined Benefit or Defined Contribution?

**Background.** When Medicare was created in the mid-1960s, it promised to deliver specific medical benefits comparable to those enjoyed by the rest of the population at that time (Butler 1998). Beneficiary premiums, out-of-pocket cost sharing, payroll taxes, and general tax revenues would finance the cost of those benefits. In some respects, Medicare today keeps that promise as well as it ever did.[6] However, Medicare costs have escalated, and one or more of those revenue sources must be tapped to keep the program's expenses and income in balance.

Health insurance programs such as Medicare, which promise to deliver a specific set of benefits, are known as defined-benefit plans. This term is borrowed from the literature on employee pensions, where it refers to a corporate promise to pay a defined retirement benefit typically based on the employee's years of service and earnings during the years immediately before retirement (Bodie and Shoven 1983). In contrast, in a defined-contribution plan the sponsor contributes to a retirement investment fund held in trust for the employee. No explicit retirement annuity or set of benefits is promised.

The terms *defined benefit* and *defined contribution*, when applied to multiple health plan settings, can be confusing. In employment-based health insurance, *defined contribution* typically means that the employer's contribution to premiums does not change from one health plan to another. An employer contribution based on the lowest-cost plan thus would be a *defined contribution* to premiums. In discussions about Medicare reform, *defined contribution* has come to mean a fixed dollar contribution that is not necessarily tied to the cost of any health plan. If we use the Medicare definition of *defined contribution*, then the defined contribution could fall below the cost of the current entitlement benefit package in some market areas.

Applied to Medicare, the defined-contribution approach implies that the government would contribute a fixed amount of money for each beneficiary. No promise would be made that this contribution would be sufficient to purchase a policy with the current (or any other specific) level of benefits.

Several arguments favor a defined-contribution approach for Medicare. First, by contributing a specified amount for the purchase of health insurance, rather than a reimbursement schedule for covered services, the government could detach the Medicare budget from the escalating cost of medical care (Butler and Moffit 1995). This reform would permit the government to limit outflows from the Medicare trust funds and the general Treasury, and thus would ensure the long-run solvency of the program.

Second, advocates argue that by combining the defined contribution with another idea—that of giving employees a choice among health insurance plans—competition for beneficiaries among plans would hold down costs more effectively than explicit regulation of prices or premiums would. As long as the government's contribution did not exceed the premium for a basic Medicare policy, beneficiaries would have to pay the marginal premiums of more expensive options out of their own pockets. Proposals that combine defined contributions and beneficiary choice are often categorized as Medicare *vouchers* (Moon and Davis 1995; Butler and Moffit 1995).[7] Among employers offering multiple health insurance plans, those making a defined contribution to premiums have lower total health insurance premiums than those subsidizing the marginal cost of more-expensive options (Dowd and Feldman 1998).

**Our Proposal.** Our proposals for Medicare reform (Dowd et al. 1992; Dowd, Feldman, and Christianson 1996; Feldman and Dowd 1998) were also based on the notion of a Medicare voucher. However, we are concerned primarily with the method of setting the voucher and less with the package of benefits being purchased. The first priority of Medicare reform should be to correct market failure. From the government's perspective, the primary source of market failure is the distorted price at which the government purchases the Medicare entitlement (the benefits to which all beneficiaries are entitled).[8]

We proposed that the government specify an initial entitlement package of benefits (possibly even the current benefit package) and solicit bids from qualified health plans to deliver that package. The government's premium contribution would be set at the lowest bid for the entitlement package of benefits received from a qualified health plan within each defined market area. Fee-for-service Medicare would be required to participate in the bidding process and would receive the same defined contribution as any other qualified health plan. This initial level of entitlement benefits and associated bids would kick off a process of obtaining an undistorted price for each level of benefits. Once the government had a process for obtaining an undistorted price for each level of entitlement benefits, the likelihood that the government would choose the efficient level for the entitlement would be vastly improved. Our proposal differs from the current entitlement in one important respect: beneficiaries maintain their right to purchase the entitlement package for only the Part B premium, but only from the most efficient health plan in the market area, not the FFS delivery system.

The effect of our proposal is illustrated in figure 7–1. The quantity of Medicare benefits is measured on the horizontal axis, and the price of benefits, on the vertical axis. The demand for Medicare benefits is labeled *DD*. Currently, benefits are bought from the inefficient FFS delivery system at prices corresponding to the *CC* supply curve. If benefits were purchased by using the bid from the most efficient health plan (labeled *EE*), the quantity of benefits would increase from $Q_c$ to $Q_e$.

It would be appealing to call our proposal a defined-benefits approach to Medicare reform because it guarantees that the benefit package is set at a given level when health plans submit their bids. Over time, however, both the demand and supply curves could change. We have already noted the discrepancy between Medicare benefits and those available in most employment-based insurance policies. In addition, Medicare must compete with government spending generally and with other entitlement programs whose needs may be more pressing than Medicare's. Changes in medical technology or an increase in the life expectancy of beneficiaries could shift the supply (cost) curve for a given package of benefits. Given these uncertainties about future demand and supply, benefits could fall or rise in the long run.

The attractiveness of our proposal does not rely on the false assur-

# FIGURE 7–1

### DEMAND AND SUPPLY OF MEDICARE ENTITLEMENT BENEFITS

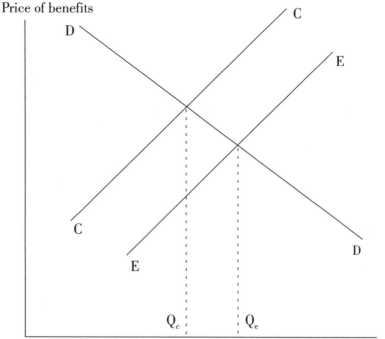

Price of benefits

D

C

E

C

E

$Q_c$

$Q_e$

Quantity of benefits

SOURCE: Authors.

ance of a permanent defined-benefit package. Instead, our proposal promotes the purchase of the efficient level of benefits at every point in time. This is the package where the demand for benefits intersects the supply price of benefits offered by the most efficient health plan.

In more general terms, the distinction between defined-benefits and defined-contribution approaches to Medicare reform is somewhat artificial and could be dropped. Furthermore, by doing so we might discard several inessential arguments and focus more clearly on the real issues facing Medicare. For example, the claim that a defined-contribution approach will ensure the solvency of Medicare is inaccurate. By definition, the present value of the Medicare deficit, plus the present value of general and earmarked taxes (including the Part B premium and out-of-pocket payments), must equal the present value of Medicare expenses. This is true whether or not the Medicare trust funds show a positive balance or, as current projections indicate, a deficit in the year 2008. It is not even clear that Medicare expenses would be more predictable if a defined contribution replaced defined benefits. The contribution formula ultimately must be determined by the political process; such a process may be every bit as complicated as determining the package of entitlement benefits. Furthermore, some proposals (Aaron and Reischauer 1995) would tie the government's Medicare contribution to the growth rate of spending by the nonelderly population. Private-sector spending growth may be even less stable than Medicare spending (especially if spending is measured by private premiums).

The real issue is that government currently purchases too few benefits at too high a price, compared with the level that would be purchased at the efficient price. A system of competitive bidding, with the government's contribution equal to the lowest bid, would guarantee that the efficient benefits would be purchased.

## Efficient Health Plan Choice in the Medicare Program

**Background.** Recently, in discussions regarding the Medicare Competitive Pricing Demonstration, the idea has been advanced that obtaining the best price from participating HMOs in the Medicare program may be less important than, or even at odds with, ensuring that the highest-risk beneficiaries are enrolled in the health plan that does the best job of caring for them.[9] The term *best job* seems to be synonymous with *most-cost-effective*. Cost-effective health plans may be able to reduce the likelihood of adverse medical events and may provide more-cost-effective treatment. Implicit in the discussions of high-risk beneficiaries and cost-effective health plans is the notion that some high-risk individuals may need to move from their current health plan to a different plan. The purpose of this section is to help frame that discussion.

Medicare has two important aspects. First, it provides health insurance to current beneficiaries and the promise of health insurance to future beneficiaries. Virtually all Americans who live long enough will become eligible for Medicare under the age entitlement. Others may become eligible as disabled or ESRD beneficiaries. That insurance function of Medicare is the focus of this section. A second important aspect of Medicare involves the redistribution of income among beneficiaries. These transfers appear to be progressive, because high-income beneficiaries contribute more to the program in payroll taxes and general tax revenues over their lifetime than low-income beneficiaries, but receive the same coverage. However, McClellan and Skinner's analysis (1997) suggests that the net transfer is, in fact, regressive. In this section, we assume that the income-redistribution part of Medicare, whatever its net effects may be, is working well, that is, reflecting the direction and degree of income redistribution desired by society. This assumption allows us to focus our attention on issues of efficiency in the beneficiary's choice of health plans.

**Consumer Risk and Health Plan Choice.** We assume that high-risk beneficiaries choose a health plan to maximize their happiness (or expected happiness). Factors contributing to the happiness associated with a specific health plan include its premium; levels of coverage (the types of services covered and the amount of point-of-purchase cost sharing); number, type, and quality of participating providers; the patient's familiarity with particular doctors; convenience factors (waiting times for appointments, office waiting times, and travel time); and the health outcomes produced by the treatment of illness and injuries.

Consider the choice between two health plans. One plan is more cost-effective than the other. We define *cost-effectiveness* as achieving the same health outcomes but at lower cost.

If the only objective were to have the high-risk beneficiaries enrolled in the cost-effective health plan, and we knew which plan that was, then only the cost-effective plan should be offered. However, as noted, beneficiaries may care about other features of health plans. Excluding the cost-ineffective health plan from the choices offered to beneficiaries would ignore beneficiaries' preferences. If beneficiaries have good information about the cost and quality of the health plans available in the market and if they are willing to pay the extra cost of cost-ineffective care, then it is inefficient to prevent them from doing so.

To achieve efficient consumer choice, we must ensure that beneficiaries face health plan premiums that reflect the difference between cost-effective and cost-ineffective care, rather than the risk of enrollees in the health plan. That is the explicit purpose of risk-adjusted payment systems.

The crucial question is, What is the relationship between the beneficiary's health risk and preference for cost-effective health plans? Two cases are of interest: high-risk beneficiaries may prefer the cost-effective plan, or they may prefer the cost-ineffective plan.

*HRHC beneficiaries prefer cost-effective health plans.* If high-risk high-cost (HRHC) beneficiaries prefer the cost-effective plan, there seems to be little to worry about. However, the distribution of enrollees across plans can be inefficient when premiums are based on the average cost of beneficiaries in the plan, rather than on the cost of individual beneficiaries. The problem is shown diagrammatically in figure 7–2.[10] We assume that two health plans—a cost-effective plan and a cost-ineffective plan—compete for market share in a population of fixed size. The population could be all employees in a firm or all Medicare beneficiaries in a given market area. The horizontal axis of figure 7–2 measures the cost-ineffective health plan's market share up to 100 percent, and the vertical axis measures dollars.

Figure 7–2 has two basic parts. The first relates to the demand for health plans, and the second, to cost. On the demand side, we hypothesize that each consumer has a willingness to pay (measured in dollars of monthly premiums) for both cost-ineffective and cost-effective health plans. Willingness to pay depends on such characteristics of the health plan as coverage, waiting times, access to providers, and perceived quality of care. Some beneficiaries may be willing to pay a large monthly premium for the cost-ineffective plan if that plan gives them access to medical specialists without a referral, for example. Other beneficiaries may be willing to pay a large premium for the cost-effective plan.

Next, we can take the difference in the consumer's willingness to pay for cost-ineffective care compared with cost-effective care. In our terminology, this relative willingness to pay is called $\Psi$. For the $i$th beneficiary, $\Psi_i = \Psi_{iCI} - \Psi_{iCE}$ , where the subscripts $CI$ and $CE$ refer to the cost-ineffective and cost-effective choices, respectively. A beneficiary would prefer to enroll in the cost-ineffective plan if $\Psi_i$ exceeds the difference in out-of-pocket premiums between the two plans.

Figure 7–2 shows the distribution of beneficiaries, ordered by their values of $\Psi$. The ordering starts with the highest value of $\Psi$, that is, the strongest preference to enroll in the cost-ineffective plan. This is followed by beneficiaries with lower values of $\Psi$, until we find some who would prefer to enroll in the cost-effective plan (negative values of $\Psi$).

On the cost side, we begin with the simple fact that enrollees in any health plan have different levels of risk. There are many levels of risk in the population, but only a few health plan choices available in any firm or Medicare market area. Most health plans ignore these interpersonal differences in risk when they set their premiums. In other words, premiums are based on the average risk enrolled by the plan, not the

# FIGURE 7–2

PREFERENCE OF HIGH-RISK BENEFICIARIES FOR COST-EFFECTIVE CARE

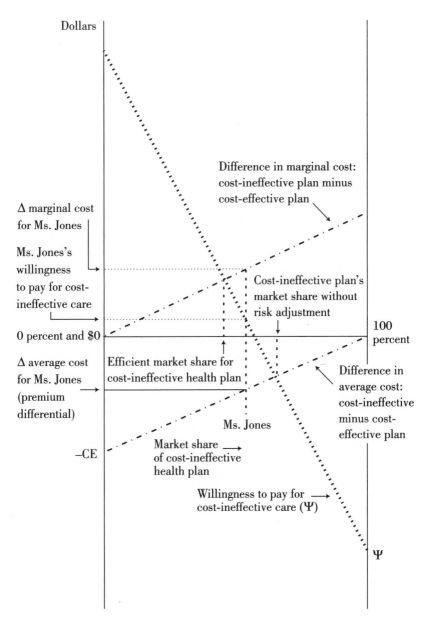

risk of each enrollee. Medicare goes one step further: it *requires* health plans to base their premiums on an average risk rather than individual risks. Medicare health plans submit what we call a local average-cost community rate—the term *local* refers to a market area, and *average-cost community rate* means that plans submit one premium for all the beneficiaries whom they expect to enroll. That premium equals the expected average cost of enrollees in the plan.

We can calculate the difference in average cost between the cost-ineffective and the cost-effective plan (as we did with willingness to pay). The line labeled "difference in average cost: cost-ineffective minus cost-effective plan" shows this difference in figure 7–2. The location of this line is a critical part of our model. In theory, consumers with a strong preference for cost-ineffective care could have either the lowest risk or the highest risk. This version of the model assumes that beneficiaries who prefer cost-ineffective care have the lowest risk (that is, high values of $\Psi$ are matched with low risk). Thus, if these beneficiaries join the cost-ineffective plan, its average cost and premium will be quite low compared with those for the remainder of the population who enroll in the cost-effective plan. The difference between the average cost of ineffective and effective health plans would be negative for this subset of enrollees. For this reason, the difference in average cost line is negative at its origin, point $-CE$.

As we move to the right in the diagram, the health risks for beneficiaries rise. Enrollment of higher-risk beneficiaries will increase the average cost (and premium) for the cost-ineffective plan. Thus, the difference in average cost becomes less negative as we move to the right. When the cost-ineffective plan has 100 percent of the market share, we assume that the last high-risk high-cost beneficiary left in the cost-effective plan has an average cost equal to that for all other beneficiaries in the cost-ineffective plan. That is why $\Delta$ average cost is zero on the right-hand side of the figure.

Under local average-cost community rating, each health plan submits a premium equal to the average cost of its enrollees. If there are no adjustments to these community rates, then each beneficiary will compare them with a willingness to pay for the cost-ineffective plan. The beneficiary will choose cost-ineffective care if $\Psi$ is greater than the premium difference for cost-ineffective care. But the market cannot be in equilibrium if any beneficiary prefers cost-ineffective care more than the premium difference. The market share of cost-ineffective care will increase until an equilibrium is reached where the $\Psi$ and the $\Delta$ average cost lines intersect. In other words, the market share of the cost-ineffective plan will increase until the last beneficiary's willingness to pay for cost-ineffective care equals the difference in average costs between the competing health plans.

To understand why the equilibrium is inefficient, we need to draw one more line in figure 7–2. This is the difference in marginal cost between the two health plans, shown by the Δ marginal cost line in figure 7–2. This line represents the difference in the cost of caring for each individual beneficiary in the two health plans as their health risk increases, in moving from left to right.

The inefficiency of equilibrium without risk adjustment can be illustrated by considering a particular beneficiary, Ms. Jones, shown on the horizontal axis. Because her willingness to pay for the cost-ineffective plan is greater than the difference in average cost for the two plans, she will join the cost-ineffective plan. However, the difference in her own cost between the two plans is more than her willingness to pay for cost-ineffective care. In other words, she is not willing to pay enough to join the cost-ineffective plan to cover her contribution to its costs. When any person is unwilling to pay for the cost of any item consumed, then consumption of this item is inefficient. In this case, Ms. Jones's consumption of the cost-ineffective plan is inefficient. The efficient outcome is for her to join the cost-effective health plan, because her willingness to pay for cost-effective care exceeds her own difference in costs between the two plans. But efficiency is thwarted by the requirement of average-cost community rating.

Under the assumptions of this model, average-cost community rating results in too few beneficiaries choosing the cost-effective health plan. The inefficiency is not due to managed care, cream skimming, profiteering, or any other popular explanation. It is due to the requirement of average-cost community rating.

Efficient choice could be achieved by dropping the average-cost community rating requirement and allowing the two plans to charge Ms. Jones her own marginal cost in each plan. This ultimate form of risk adjustment, individual experience rating, guarantees an efficient allocation of beneficiaries to health plans by having beneficiaries face premium differentials that reflect only efficiency (cost) differences in the two plans, not differences in risk. Of course, individual experience rating may result in higher-risk beneficiaries facing higher out-of-pocket premium differentials. That may be considered unfair, but it is not inefficient, unless there are incomplete markets for long-term risk protection.

Another risk-adjustment approach to resolving the problem of inefficient allocation is to adjust the difference in out-of-pocket premiums between the two plans faced by all beneficiaries to reflect marginal-cost–pricing, rather than average-cost–pricing (Feldman and Dowd 1994). This resolution can be achieved by increasing the employer's (or government's) premium contribution to the cost-effective plan. Using either method (individual experience rating or out-of-pocket premium adjustments) could, in theory, achieve the efficient allocation of beneficiaries to the cost-effective health plan shown in figure 7–2. The information requirements for these two approaches are quite different, however. The experience-rating approach requires only that health plans know the cost of beneficiaries in each risk category. Marginal-cost community rating also requires knowledge of consumer preferences for cost-ineffective care (that is, the slope of the $\Psi$ line).

This theory justifies some type of risk adjustment to achieve an efficient distribution of beneficiaries among cost-effective and cost-ineffective health plans. It is an appealing theory, because it suggests that too few beneficiaries are enrolled in cost-effective health plans, and something can be done to fix the problem. The theory has only one difficulty: empirical evidence refutes the assumption that beneficiaries who prefer cost-ineffective care have the lowest risk. HRHC beneficiaries, on average, are much more likely to prefer cost-ineffective care. This evidence has important implications for the analysis.

*High-risk beneficiaries prefer cost-ineffective health plans.* The most common comparisons of cost-effective and cost-ineffective health plans compare health maintenance organizations to traditional fee-for-service health plans. Four points stand out in those reviews. First, HMOs reduce the utilization of services and spending by enrollees (Miller and Luft 1994). Second, as noted, careful studies based on chart reviews and analysis of SEER data suggest that the quality of care in Medicare HMOs either equals or exceeds care in the FFS sector. Third, HMOs generally enroll lower-risk beneficiaries than FFS health plans (Brown et al. 1993). Fourth, in many parts of the country, Medicare HMOs charge no out-of-pocket premium (beyond the Part B premium). Many of those "free" HMOs offer generous supplementary benefits. Thus, many high-risk beneficiaries apparently are willing to forgo generous free benefits to remain in the FFS sector.

If high-risk beneficiaries prefer cost-ineffective care, then the slope of the $\Psi$ line in figure 7–2 must be reversed. Instead of sloping down (to the right), it must slope up. The revised diagram is shown in figure 7–3. In figure 7–3, the horizontal axis measures the market share of the cost-effective health plan rather than the cost-ineffective plan. Otherwise, the diagram remains unchanged, because the average and marginal cost lines still are oriented toward increasingly higher-risk beneficiaries as we move from left to right.

Now, the situation is quite different. Average-cost community rating without risk adjustment produces an equilibrium with too many beneficiaries in cost-effective care rather than too few. Ms. Jones is willing to pay more than her own cost differential to enroll in cost-ineffective care but less than the difference in premiums resulting from average-cost community rating.

Individual experience rating would restore efficiency by allowing Ms. Jones to pay her own $\Delta$ marginal cost for cost-ineffective care. Alternatively, larger government contributions to the cost-ineffective health plan would produce the efficient (lower) market share for the cost-effective plan, as shown in figure 7–3.

**Poor Information.** In addition to the requirement of average-cost community rating, poor consumer information about other health plan characteristics (such as the costs of different health plans, waiting times for appointments or office waits, differences in health outcomes, the number and type of in-network providers) could produce inefficient choices. For example, cost-effective health plans could reduce the patient's time costs by reducing unnecessary physician office visits. Cost-effective care also could reduce the risks associated with unnecessary tests and hospitalizations. High-risk beneficiaries could be misinformed about these effects. If poor information is the primary problem, the solution is to produce and disseminate better information, as long as the benefits of doing so outweigh the costs.

Suppose that the government has better information than beneficiaries do on the quality of care. The only legitimate reason for withholding information from consumers is that the cost of dissemination outweighs the benefits. Believing that beneficiaries would not act on the information if it were disseminated is not a legitimate reason to withhold it. Nor is it efficient to alter out-of-pocket premiums to manipulate health plan choices if beneficiaries fail to act on information. Beneficiaries probably have a reason for their decision; replacing individual consumer choice with centralized decisionmaking is likely to produce substantial inefficiency. Altering out-of-pocket premiums because of in-

## FIGURE 7–3
### Preference of High-Risk Beneficiaries for Cost-Ineffective Care

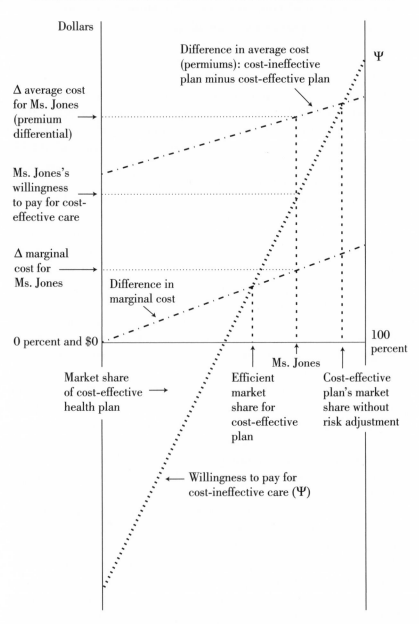

Source: Authors.

formation that consumers have in hand merely introduces another distortion into the prices that consumers face. Stories about the government (or employers) being able to use the information more effectively than consumers must be told carefully.

## Summary

Policymakers may find it frustrating that high-risk beneficiaries choose cost-ineffective health plans. The apparent solution—moving high-risk beneficiaries into more cost-effective health plans—should be pursued carefully, however. Average-cost community rating can lead to inefficient health plan choice. Adjusting for the difference in premiums that beneficiaries face for risk, by allowing health plans to experience-rate, will restore efficient choice, but the premium differentials might be higher for some beneficiaries than others. Premium differentials can be kept the same for everyone and achieve efficient market shares for health plans only if the government contributes different amounts to different health plans so that the beneficiary's premium differential equals the difference in marginal costs of beneficiaries at the efficient equilibrium market share.

In contrast, we propose that the government set a level dollar contribution equal to the lowest-priced qualified health plan in the market area. If it were possible to know both the marginal cost of enrollees in different health plans and the location of the $\Psi$ line, then we would recommend marginal-cost community rating instead. Without that information, however, we must choose among less desirable alternatives. The desirable features of the low-bid contribution are (1) it provides the greatest incentive for health plans to compete and (2) the low-bid contribution appears likely to produce the less expensive, if not the lesser, of the two evils, given the choice of too few or too many people in cost-effective health plans.

If out-of-pocket premiums are corrected for risk, predicting the new equilibrium distribution of enrollees may be difficult. If high-risk beneficiaries prefer cost-effective health plans, then the market share of cost-effective health plans will increase with risk adjustment. If high-risk beneficiaries prefer cost-ineffective health plans, however, the market share of cost-effective health plans will decrease with risk adjustment. Evidence from the Medicare program favors the latter prediction. Rather than being at odds with the objective of moving high-risk beneficiaries into cost-effective care, a defined contribution to premiums without risk adjustment may actually move more high-risk beneficiaries into cost-effective care than risk-adjusting out-of-pocket premiums.

If the choice of cost-ineffective health plans results from poor information, then the allocation of beneficiaries to health plans under any payment system could be inefficient. The benchmark solution for poor information—against which other proposals should be judged—is to generate better information and put it in the hands of beneficiaries. Only if the costs of dissemination outweigh the expected benefits should government consider altering out-of-pocket premiums because of information that it believes is superior to beneficiaries' information.

The concept of manipulating out-of-pocket premiums to move beneficiaries (or employees) into cost-effective care is questionable for several reasons. First, it is unlikely that any single health plan is uniformly more cost-effective than its competitors for all types of medical conditions. Second, even if a "planner" could identify a health plan that consistently outperformed all others on some cost-effectiveness measure, and we observed beneficiaries choosing other health plans, we still could not conclude that those choices were inefficient in an economic sense. Economic efficiency does not depend on the preferences of planners, no matter how well-intentioned the planners. Efficiency depends on the preferences of consumers, who may have made choices based on factors other than the planner's measure of cost-effective care. If the planner was better informed than the consumer, one still would have to explain why the better information was not given to consumers, rather than used by the planner to manipulate out-of-pocket premiums.

Planners who attempt to manipulate out-of-pocket premiums are likely to find themselves facing an unpleasant choice. They could attempt to achieve the relative efficiency of marginal-cost community rating by using risk adjustments to the average-cost premiums submitted by health plans. That adjustment would probably result in out-of-pocket premium differentials between cost-effective and cost-ineffective health plans that would be narrower than the unadjusted premium differentials. The likely result is that more beneficiaries would remain in higher-cost, cost-ineffective health plans. Alternatively, the planner could attempt to widen the out-of-pocket premium differential between cost-effective and cost-ineffective health plans to encourage migration to cost-effective plans. That adjustment would probably result in increased economic inefficiency, because consumers would be moved from health plans for which they willingly would pay their true marginal cost of joining.

The Medicare program faces severe challenges. Unless Medicare in its current form is to be a one-time gift to current retirees (and this is a defensible proposal), it faces an intolerable problem of intergenerational fairness, and the program's revenue and expenditure streams will need dramatic alteration. Attempting to remedy the situation through increased tax revenue alone is probably infeasible and would raise a new set of intergenerational fairness problems. The optimal path to greater fairness is greater efficiency, based on a new way to set the government's contribution to premiums. We recommend a contribution method that is both a defined contribution (constant across all plans) and a defined benefit (the Medicare entitlement package of benefits, purchased from the lowest-cost qualified health plan in each market area).[11]

In a world constrained by average-cost community rating, we also favor implementation of risk-adjusted payments to health plans, as long as the development of that system does not impede progress toward a competitive pricing system for determining the government's contribution to premiums. Because high-risk beneficiaries seem to prefer the FFS sector, adjusting payments to Medicare HMOs by risks, even in a truly competitive pricing system that includes the FFS sector as a bidder, is likely to result in more high-risk beneficiaries choosing the FFS sector, which may offer less cost-effective care. If the high-risk beneficiaries' FFS care is based on reasonably good information, and if the beneficiaries are willing to pay the risk-adjusted marginal cost of the FFS sector out of their own pockets, then their choice of a cost-inefficient health plan would be economically efficient.

## Notes

1. These projections use the trustees' intermediate assumptions.

2. Increasing the age of eligibility may be particularly regressive, since life expectancy is positively related to income (McClellan and Skinner 1997).

3. The regressiveness of those cuts could be addressed by targeted financial aid, however, such as the Qualified Medicare Beneficiary (QMB) and Special Low-Income Medicare Beneficiary (SLMB) Programs.

4. Under the payment system established by the Balanced Budget Act of 1997, the savings could increase in high-payment areas, but costs also have increased in low-payment areas. The net result is budget neutrality.

5. In our book *Competitive Pricing for Medicare*, we provide solutions to the problems of adequate capacity in the lowest-priced plans, predatory pricing, and other concerns about a low-bid contribution.

6. However, the medical insurance benefits enjoyed by the general population have outpaced Medicare in two areas: private health insurance plans for the nonelderly almost always cover prescription drugs, and they provide protection against catastrophic medical bills up to $1 million or $2 million. Medicare has neither benefit.

7. The analogy in employee pensions is workers' choice of how their defined contributions are invested.

8. Beneficiaries not only face distorted prices but also have relatively little information about the quality, quantity, and price of benefits offered by competing health plans in their market area.

9. *Highest cost* is not synonymous with *highest risk*. A high-risk person has a high probability of experiencing an adverse health event but has not yet done so. A high-cost person has already experienced the adverse health event, and thus it is known with certainty that he will have higher than average costs in the current period. A person can be both high cost and high risk. A person with diabetes may have high costs of care and also be a higher risk of heart disease, for example.

10. This diagram has been used in Feldman and Dowd 1982, Dowd and Feldman 1998, Ellis and McGuire 1987, and Cutler and Zeckhauser 1998.

11. Cutler and Zeckhauser (1998) argue that low-risk consumers may be willing to subsidize the premiums of higher-cost health plans to reduce the premium differential that they would face if they should decide to switch to a higher-cost plan when they become ill. This argument deserves careful consideration.

# References

Aaron, Henry J., and Robert D. Reischauer. 1995. "The Medicare Reform Debate: What Is the Next Step?" *Health Affairs* 14 (4) (winter): 8–30.

Board of Trustees of the Hospital Insurance Trust Fund. 1995, 1998. *Annual Report of the Board of Trustees of the Hospital Insurance Trust Fund.* Washington, D.C.: Government Printing Office.

Board of Trustees of the Supplemental Medical Insurance Trust Fund. 1995, 1998. *Annual Report of the Board of Trustees of the Supplemental Medical Insurance Trust Fund.* Washington, D.C.: Government Printing Office.

Bodie, Zvi, and John B. Shoven. 1983. "Introduction." In *Financial Aspects of the United States Pension System*, edited by Zvi Bodie and John B. Shoven. Chicago: University of Chicago Press.

Brown, R. S., D. G. Clement, J. W. Hill, S. M. Retchin, and J. W. Bergeron.

1993. "Do Health Maintenance Organizations Work for Medicare?" *Health Care Financing Review* 15 (1) (fall): 7–24.

Butler, Stuart A. 1998. "The Contract and Medicare Reform." In *Medicare: Preparing for the Challenges of the Twenty-First Century*, edited by Robert D. Reischauer, Stuart Butler, and Judith R. Lave. Washington, D.C.: Brookings Institution Press.

Butler, Stuart A., and Robert E. Moffit. 1995. "The FEHBP as a Model for a New Medicare Program." *Health Affairs* 14 (4) (winter): 47–61.

Carlisle, D. M., A. L. Siu, E. B. Keeler, K. L. Lahn, L. V. Rubenstein, and R. H. Brook. 1994. "Do HMOs Provide Better Care for Older Patients with Acute Myocardial Infarction?" In *HMOs and the Elderly*, edited by Harold Luft. Ann Arbor, Mich.: Health Administration Press.

Cutler, David M., and Sarah J. Reber. 1998. "Paying for Health Insurance: The Tradeoff between Competition and Adverse Selection." *Quarterly Journal of Economics* 113 (2) (May): 433–66.

Cutler, David M., and Richard J. Zeckhauser. 1998. "Adverse Selection in Health Insurance." In *Frontiers in Health Policy Research*, vol. 1, edited by Alan Garber. Cambridge: MIT Press.

Dowd, Bryan E., Jon C. Christianson, Roger D. Feldman, Catherine Wisner, and John Klein. 1992. "Issues regarding Health Plan Payments under Medicare and Recommendations for Reform." *Milbank Quarterly* 70 (no. 3): 423–53.

Dowd, Bryan E., and Roger D. Feldman. 1998. "Employer Premium Contributions and Health Care Costs." In *Managed Care and Changing Health Care Markets*, edited by Michael A. Morrisey. Washington, D.C.: AEI Press.

Dowd, Bryan E., Roger Feldman, and Jon Christianson. 1996. *Competitive Pricing for Medicare*. Washington, D.C.: AEI Press.

Ellis, Randall P., and Thomas G. McGuire. 1987. "Setting Capitation Payments in Markets for Health Services." *Health Care Financing Review* 8 (4): 55–64.

Feldman, Roger, and Bryan E. Dowd. 1982. "Simulation of a Health Insurance Market with Adverse Selection." *Operations Research* 30 (6): 1027–42.

Feldman, Roger D., and Bryan E. Dowd. 1994. "Risk Adjustment in the Theory of Managed Competition." Division of Health Services Research and Policy, University of Minnesota.

Feldman, Roger, and Bryan Dowd. 1998. "Structuring Choice under Medicare." In *Medicare: Preparing for the Challenges of the Twenty-First*

*Century*, edited by Robert D. Reischauer, Stuart Butler, and Judith R. Lave. Washington, D.C.: Brookings Institution Press.

McClellan, Mark, and Jonathan Skinner. 1997. "The Incidence of Medicare." National Bureau of Economic Research Working Paper 6013.

Miller, R. H., and H. S. Luft. 1994. "Managed Care Plan Performance since 1980: A Literature Analysis." *Journal of the American Medical Association* 271 (19):1512–19.

Moon, Marilyn, and Karen Davis. 1995. "Preserving and Strengthening Medicare." *Health Affairs* 14 (4) (winter): 31–46.

Retchin, S. M., D. G. Clement, and R. S. Brown. 1994. "Care of Patients Hospitalized with Strokes under the Medicare Risk Program." In *HMOs and the Elderly*, edited by Harold Luft. Ann Arbor, Mich.: Health Administration Press.

Riley, Gerald F., Arnold L. Potosky, James D. Lubitz, and Martin L. Brown. 1994. "Stage of Cancer at Diagnosis for Medicare HMO and Fee-for-Service Enrollees." *American Journal of Public Health* 84 (10) (October): 1598–1604.

# 8

---

# The FEHBP as a
# Model for Reform

## Walton Francis

The purpose of this analysis is to examine the Federal Employees
Health Benefits Program (FEHBP) as a potential model for Medicare reform. Is the program a good model, a bad model, or irrel-
evant? Which Medicare problems might it solve, and which exacerbate
or leave unchanged?

These questions are relevant for three reasons. First, it is widely
agreed that Medicare is both an antiquated and inadequate insurance
program, and likely to become insolvent in about a decade. Second, the
FEHBP is widely recognized as a program that has performed well and
avoided many difficulties by relying on competitive choice among private-sector health insurance plans rather than legislative and bureaucratic fiat for its evolution, design, and workings. Third, the bipartisan
Medicare commission appointed by the president and Congress considered a "premium-support" reform option proposed by the commission
cochairmen, Senator John Breaux and Representative Bill Thomas, that
is explicitly "patterned after the Federal Employees Health Benefits
Program . . . that provides health insurance for nine million federal
employees, retirees, and dependents" (National Bipartisan Commis-

sion 1999b). Of course, this is not a new idea. The first Medicare proposal modeled substantially after the FEHBP came from Alain Enthoven (1980). His proposal, remarkably similar to Breaux-Thomas, had an even catchier title, "Freedom of Choice," referring to the proposal's empowerment of beneficiaries to choose plans with lower premiums or better benefits. More recently, Stuart Butler and Robert Moffit of the Heritage Foundation made a similar proposal (Butler and Moffit 1995), as did the American Medical Association (1995).

This chapter first describes the workings of the FEHBP. Then, it provides information on overall FEHBP performance, particularly in comparison with Medicare performance, and identifies the FEHBP design features that should be considered, or avoided, in reforming Medicare. For example, plan-by-plan flexibility in benefit design has been central to FEHBP success. Variations in benefits among plans are an essential factor (along with cost competition and service quality) in meeting short-term consumer needs and in stimulating long-term reforms. Freezing benefits in a one-size-fits-all design that can be changed only by the political process is one of Medicare's greatest weaknesses. The FEHBP's flexibility has come at some cost in risk selection, but techniques already used by Medicare could eliminate undesirable risk selection. (As I argue below, having consumers pay extra for better benefits and sorting themselves into plans that offer particular benefits are desirable forms of risk selection.)

What the FEHBP model cannot do is halt the seemingly inexorable dynamics of more Americans turning sixty-five, of increasing longevity among the elderly, and of rising technology-driven medical care costs (Board of Trustees 1999). This model depends on and cannot perform better than the underlying medical care market—although it can influence that market to perform better and save money. But if the underlying costs continue to grow exponentially, no reform model can solve the long-term problem.

Using the FEHBP as a model is, to some, a thinly disguised attempt to shift costs from taxpayers to the elderly. One opponent said that allotting a lump sum to each Medicare beneficiary and having individuals negotiate with insurance companies would be "throwing people to the wolves" (John Firman, president, National Council on Aging, quoted in "Some Think Tanks, Industry Groups Urge GOP to Convert Medicare to a Voucherlike System," *Wall Street Journal,* July 13, 1995). In this context, *defined benefit* is seen as a generous measure to preserve guarantees, *defined contribution* as a mean-spirited attempt to increase the cost burden on the elderly, and *vouchers* as a symbol of unconstrained competition.

In fact, the FEHBP model is essentially neutral. It is compatible with benefit reductions and increases in beneficiary premiums and cost-sharing, or with benefit increases and reduced premiums and costs. The model provides one way to introduce prescription drug coverage into Medicare. The FEHBP model also provides a way to modify cost-sharing by beneficiaries in a relatively painless and gradual way. Design choices would determine whether the reformed program would be more or less generous to each of the various parties involved: payroll taxpayers, income taxpayers, beneficiaries, private-sector pension plans, states (as Medicaid payers of premiums and deductibles for low-income elderly), and providers. Potentially, the FEHBP model could reduce the costs to all affected interests through improved cost-reduction.

## How the FEHBP Works

**Background.** The FEHBP is unique among government health insurance programs in relying primarily on the private market for almost all functions, including many policy decisions on benefits design. During World War II, private employer health insurance grew rapidly because the government's wage-control program exempted health insurance. But the government eschewed this loophole for its own employees, and insurance plans sponsored by unions and employee associations grew up to fill this void. By 1959, the executive branch proposed a system under which the government would determine benefits and payments in a single fee-for-service plan that all employees would join. This proposal was modeled after large-employer practices. Because unions and employees did not want to abandon their own plans, a compromise grandfathered existing plans to compete with two governmentwide plans in an annual open season (Anderson and May 1971). New entrants to health maintenance organizations (HMOs) would be allowed but new fee-for-service entrants would not. In 1980, Congress enacted a time-limited opportunity for new fee-for-service plans affiliated with employee organizations to join. Of the half dozen that accepted this offer, only one survives.

To allow multiple plans to coexist, the annual open season lets employees switch from plan to plan and, in a deliberately planned invitation to risk selection, from high to low options within the same plan. Preexisting condition exclusions are banned. Any employee, no matter how ill, may join any plan. Competition forces plans to respond to consumer preferences for benefits, service, and economy.

**The Mechanics of the Program.** About 300 health insurance plans participate in the FEHBP. Most of them are HMOs that cover self-defined geographic areas. In 1999, every federal employee or annuitant could choose from about a dozen fee-for-service (FFS)/preferred-provider (PPO) options, and most could choose from almost two dozen options, depending on the number of local HMOs.

Choices include nationwide plans sponsored by Blue Cross/Blue Shield and by unions and employee associations and almost 300 HMOs. The nationwide plans are all nominally fee-for-service, but virtually all have evolved into preferred provider plans over the last decade. Employees are free to join most union and association plans. At most they must pay annual dues, generally near $30. However, some plans do restrict enrollment. There are almost 3 million covered employees and more than 1 1/2 million covered annuitants, for a total of 4 1/2 million contracts and some 9 million covered lives. Employees are also free to switch among plans at certain other times—for instance, if they marry or move out of an HMO's service area. (More details on the programs can be found in Merck 1999.)

Many employees and annuitants are enrolled in plans that are much more expensive than average. In each open season almost all these individuals can reduce premium costs while maintaining or even improving benefits. Most do not change plans: only 5 percent of enrollees switch plans in most open seasons.

**Implementation.** The Office of Personnel Management (OPM) sets financial, administrative, and benefit terms and conditions for every plan in the program. Most standards are informal and subject to negotiation. After negotiation, insurance companies and OPM agree each year on contracts setting forth both benefits and premium costs.

The mechanics of enrollment are handled by hundreds of government personnel offices for active employees and by OPM directly for annuitants. Agency payroll computers and OPM retirement computers deduct for each plan. Payments for both employee and government shares are transferred electronically to OPM for plan payment. Annuitant procedures are handled almost entirely by mail.

The program relies on strong mechanisms to protect enrollees: clear and complete information on benefits and limitations, open season, plans that are available in the open market and not limited to federal enrollees, and an independent appeal process.

**OPM Role.** The Office of Personnel Management operates in a fiduciary capacity in administering the program. Its antennae focus on issues such as the status of the trust funds, the status of government and plan reserves, trends in the health care market, the effects of plans' benefit decisions on premiums, and the financial viability, actuarial value, general benefit structure, specific benefits, general competence, clarity of brochures, and appeal procedures of each plan.

In general, OPM operates in a management-by-exception role. If a plan is not doing something drastically wrong, OPM is passive and accepting. OPM is, in essence, a referee with limited responsibility. However, in some areas OPM has vigorously led the programs—such as providing information to enrollees to make open season work through informed choices.

OPM administers the program with approximately 150 government employees, compared with the thousands of persons who administer Medicare, TriCare/CHAMPUS (Civilian Health and Medical Program of the Uniformed Services), and Medicaid. Almost half the OPM effort is devoted to processing appeals of plan coverage decisions, rather than to policysetting and direct administration.

**Premiums.** The total premium for each plan for a given calendar year is calculated from the estimated costs for that year, as forecast by the plan and reviewed and agreed to by the government. Various standards of reasonableness are the sole controls or limits on this estimate. For community-rated plans, the government asks that the plan give the government the best group rate available to any employer. All fee-for-service plans and some HMOs are experience-rated. Experience-rating covers about two-thirds of all enrollees.

The government pays a set amount toward the total premium of each participating plan, based on a percentage of the weighted average premium for all plans. As costs rise or fall, the government contribution reacts proportionally. For calendar 1999 the maximum government contribution amount is about $1,870 annually for a self-only enrollment and $4,170 for a family of any size. The enrollee pays the rest. Under standard economic theory regarding employee compensation, the enrollee pays the entire amount. The government share is a fiction with one practical effect: the government share is paid in tax-free dollars and the enrollee share in before-tax dollars.

More precisely, for General Schedule employees and retirees, the government pays 75 percent of the total premium cost up to a maximum contribution at the amounts above. Thus, a plan with a total premium cost of $2,400 for self-only would have a government contribution of $1,800; the enrollee would pay $600. For a plan with a total premium cost of $3,700, the government and the enrollee would each pay about half.

The enrollee share of premiums varies widely. In 1999, the GS employee share ranged from about $500 to more than $3,000 for individuals and from about $1,000 to more than $6,000 for families. Why? First, plans vary in the kinds of enrollees attracted. Smaller coinsurance or larger provider networks tend to attract families who expect higher expenses. These plans face higher costs that must be made up by higher premiums. Premiums reflecting these higher costs exceed the value of the benefits compared with plans that attract lower-risk enrollees (Merlis 1999). On average, enrollees in HMOs are about six years younger than those in fee-for-service plans (Thorpe forthcoming). Risk selection has been substantial in some fee-for-service plans, as discussed below.

Further, plans offer varying benefits. Variations include different coverage, coinsurance, and deductibles. Some deductibles apply to all services. Others apply only to hospital or prescription drug costs. Some plans have three deductibles. Some benefit variations have a major effect on the value of a plan's benefits. Deductibles have an almost dollar-for-dollar effect on plan premium.

Also, plans vary in their management of health care costs. A well-run HMO might reduce the frequency and length of hospital stays by 25 percent or more compared with traditional fee-for-service insurance. Plans vary in their effectiveness in bargaining with providers. And cost-sharing creates incentives to reduce waste. Large deductibles discourage unnecessary visits, while 100 percent reimbursement encourages overuse of services. Reflecting both risk selection and plan management, fee-for-service plans have a self-only total premium for 1999 averaging about $2,720; in contrast, HMOs average only about $2,330 (unpublished tables available from the author). The total cost difference is even greater, because most HMOs have no deductibles.

Last, the government's formula for the share of its total premium magnifies the percentage differences in what enrollees pay. The enrollee pays all cost of any premium amount above the government's share. This employee share is far higher for the more expensive plans.

Thus, enrollees pay modestly for insurance from a well-run plan but more for a plan's inefficiencies, its unusually generous benefits, its greater provider access, or its large share of high-risk enrollees. The ability to switch among plans gives enrollees a major tool for obtaining the best deal.

**Premium Management.** Bids of all participating plans for a year determine the government contribution. OPM generally accepts these bids. Several factors influence OPM decisions to intervene selectively in benefit and premium proposals from the plans. First, OPM has an interest in ensuring that the plan remains solvent at least for the contract year. In some cases, this has led the plan to propose, and OPM to accept, premiums that are not actuarily "fair" but that ensure solvency until the plan exits the system.

Second, OPM has an interest in keeping premiums low, on behalf of both enrollees and the federal budget. The agency has a strong incentive to meddle in benefit decisions for the larger plans, despite the fact that enrollees pay all marginal costs once the government contribution is set. Moreover, fairness virtually forces OPM to treat plans equally in what it allows, encourages, or prohibits.

Third, OPM has an interest in promoting good benefits for its employees. In the past, a number of fee-for-service plans had grossly inadequate prescription drug coverage. Over time, OPM has pressured the less-adequate plans to improve coverage. This position has premium implications and, hence, budgetary implications for both the federal government and enrollee wallets. OPM can trade off the competing objectives of frugality and beneficence.

Changes in plan costs for existing benefit packages have a dollar-for-dollar effect on government costs. If Blue Cross and every other plan keep existing benefit packages intact but payments to providers rise by 5 percent, the next year's total premium, government contribution, and employee share will all rise by 5 percent. Thus, each year's premiums and the allocation of costs are driven by the health insurance market. In this respect, OPM is a passive price-taker—getting the best deal that it can but, as any other purchaser, accepting the dictates of a more or less competitive market.

**Benefits.** All plans must offer a core of comparable benefits. In contractual bargaining, OPM seeks to limit variations in the actuarial value. But, on the margin, benefits are not identical among the plans. Most fee-for-service plans have a deductible of several hundred dollars; most

HMOs have no deductible at all. Only some plans provide mail-order prescription drugs, chiropractic coverage, and dental coverage. Almost all fee-for-service plans vary cost-sharing, depending on whether preferred providers are used.

The statute governing the FEHBP contains only one paragraph on benefits. What ensures that each plan will cover major types of benefits adequately and without significant loopholes? First and foremost, the plans themselves do not operate in a vacuum. They are ongoing businesses in an environment in which health insurance plans typically cover (for example) hospital costs without significant exceptions or loopholes. The plans are subject to market pressures. A plan that significantly departed from benefits expected by enrollees and available in other plans would rapidly lose enrollment. Short-run gains from benefit loopholes are possible, but over time the plan could not survive.

FEHBP benefits have significantly improved over time. From 1983 to 1992, estimated out-of-pocket costs for self-only enrollees in HMO plans went from 22 percent to 12 percent of total medical and dental cost and, for those in fee-for-service plans, from 33 percent to 22 percent (Francis 1993a, b). Benefits have improved even more for enrollees willing to use preferred providers. In 1992 the Blue Cross Standard Option, the largest plan in the program, required enrollees to pay 25 percent of usual, customary, and reasonable charges for outpatient care after a $250 deductible. In 1999, a reformed Blue Cross Plan requires enrollees to pay only $12 after a $200 deductible, provided that they use preferred providers. HMO benefits have improved less because they were so good to start with.

A crucial aspect of benefit variation is that plans can experiment and evolve. Thus, in designing prescription-drug benefits, plans can use almost any combination of benefits and procedures to hold down costs while meeting consumer acceptance. These include a drug deductible, the rate of coinsurance or amount of copayment, lower copayments for generic drugs, pharmacies designated as preferred providers, and the use of mail order.

Similar, though fewer, variables are used for hospital, medical, and other expenses. Each plan decides whether to charge a separate hospital deductible and whether to waive such a deductible for admission after an accident. Some plans charge coinsurance for hospital stays; some do not.

These deductibles and coinsurance rates are tied, in turn, to decisions on the catastrophic stop-loss limit. Where the catastrophic limit is low, the plan is more likely to be willing to impose charges on hospital visits, because the enrollees' cost exposure is limited.

**Reimbursement.** Nothing in FEHBP law or regulation prescribes any particular method of reimbursement. Historically, HMOs have tended to use capitated approaches to outpatient care. Fee-for-service plans once relied primarily on usual, customary, and reasonable methodologies and, in some cases, on fee schedules that were not negotiated with physicians. Today, fee-for-service plans rely primarily on fee schedules negotiated with providers, similar to those used by HMOs. Both historically and at present, there have been no uniform payment methods across plans. Plans simply cut the best deals they can in the health care marketplace. By both fostering and relying on the changes in the private market, the FEHBP has evolved with the managed-care revolution of the 1990s.

**Provider Access.** The FEHBP has not set programwide terms and conditions regarding providers or reimbursement. Historically, the Blue Cross plans have paid better for participating providers who agree to accept a fixed rate set at a lower level than many would otherwise charge. More recently, this plan has added preferred providers who accept an even lower rate (about one-half of physicians, hospitals, and pharmacies are "preferred" under Blue Cross). Meanwhile, reimbursement to the few providers who are neither preferred nor participating has been reduced and relies on a parsimonious fee schedule borrowed from Medicare. HMOs historically have used several models, including employee providers, affiliated group practices, and individual practice associations. The numbers and kinds of arrangements are almost as diverse as the number of plans. OPM has encouraged point-of-service (POS) or opt-out arrangements recently, but fewer than one in ten HMOs have adopted these.

Plan decisions on provider access interact with decisions on reimbursement and also benefit design. For example, the decision to use mail-order pharmacies has concerned both providers and patients, particularly those elderly accustomed to a Medicare coordination benefit allowing 100 percent coverage of drugs at local pharmacies. Several years ago, the Blue Cross addition of a preferential mail-order benefit created great controversy. The state of Maryland enacted a statute to prohibit mail-order discounts. Although the law had no effect on the FEHBP Blue Cross plan—which is exempt from state regulation—the

Kaiser plan headquartered in Maryland was forced to end reduced copayments for its mail-order program.

**Geography.** Almost all fee-for-service plans operate nationally and with a single premium. HMOs operate locally; they typically cover a metropolitan area but sometimes include many counties or an entire state. The FEHBP statute does not allow any geographic distinction in premiums. Thus, the government contribution is the same everywhere, in both high-cost and low-cost areas. This uniformity is arguably a major strength. When FEHBP premiums are averaged across all plans in a service area, there is no major difference in the cost of providing HMO care across most of the country (Schmid 1995). Any differences may reflect the strengths and weaknesses of plans that are relatively dominant in particular areas. As a consequence, geographic distortions of consumer decisions are relatively attenuated and arise largely because the fee-for-service plans are not allowed to vary premiums by geographic area (Thorpe forthcoming). The FEHBP has avoided the major geographic distortions that have plagued the Medicare program, have dominated the distributive politics of Medicare (Vladek 1999), and have penalized HMOs in areas with spuriously estimated costs.

**Costs.** The FEHBP uses market competition as the essential mechanism to control costs. Though large, the program does not have enough market share to rely on monopsony power. Furthermore, cost controls (for example, procedure-by-procedure limits on payments, as used in Medicare) would be antithetical to the nature of the program. If a particular method were prescribed for payment for prescription drugs, then much flexibility in benefit design and evolution would be gone.

Relying on market forces has both short- and long-run implications. The long run is addressed below in comparing performance with Medicare. The effects of a competitive open season provide dramatic evidence of the short run. Each fall OPM publishes the enrollment-weighted average premium for the forthcoming year, under the assumption that enrollment remains the same. During the open season, about 5 percent of enrollees change plans; some select more-expensive plans, but most switch to relatively lower-cost plans. The results (table 8–1) show almost a 1 percent saving on average.

In earlier years, when insurance costs were rising much faster, open season savings were even larger. In theory, such effects might reflect risk selection rather than real savings, with migration each year

TABLE 8–1

PREMIUM SAVINGS FROM OPEN SEASON, 1994–1998

(in percent)

| Year | Before Open Season | Open Season Result | Difference |
|------|--------------------|--------------------|------------|
| 1994 | 3.0 | 2.7 | –.3 |
| 1995 | –3.4 | –3.9 | –.5 |
| 1996 | .4 | –.2 | –.6 |
| 1997 | 2.4 | 3.1 | +.7 |
| 1998 | 8.5 | 5.4 | –3.1 |
| Average | 2.2 | 1.4 | –.8 |

SOURCE: Annual OPM press releases and author. A similar calculation appears in National Bipartisan Commission 1999a.

tending to raise premiums in the next (Merck 1999). In fact, risk-selection effects are minimal, as shown by inspection of migration patterns and the long-term analysis below. Savings from plan-switching behavior might be much larger if the underlying premium formulas provided greater rewards to enrollees, and if Medicare-participating annuitants were not insulated from the cost-benefit calculus faced by employees. In practice, the government usually recoups 75 percent of the premium difference when a lower-priced plan is selected, particularly for self-enrollments. (This issue is analyzed in detail in Thorpe forthcoming.)

## Comparative Medicare and FEHBP Performance

Risk selection is the only area of Medicare superiority—using methods that the FEHBP could easily adopt. "The FEHBP has outperformed Medicare every which way—in containment of costs, both to consumers and to the government, in benefit . . . innovation and modernization, and in consumer satisfaction" (Cain 1999).

**Cost Performance.** The program consistently surpasses Medicare's performance in holding down program costs. With simple ten-year rolling averages for comparison, FEHBP's rate of increase in average benefits paid per enrollee is more than one percentage point less than Medicare (table 8–2).

## TABLE 8–2
### INCREASE IN AVERAGE COSTS PER ENROLLEE, 1995–1999
(in percent)

| Final Year of Calculation | Average Ten-Year Medicare Increase | Average Ten-Year FEHBP Increase | Difference |
|---|---|---|---|
| 1995 | 7.7 | 9.5 | 1.8 |
| 1996 | 7.9 | 7.3 | –.6 |
| 1997 | 8.2 | 7.0 | –1.2 |
| 1998 | 7.8 | 6.1 | –1.7 |
| 1999 | 7.4 | 5.8 | –1.6 |

SOURCE: Congress 1998; author. The National Bipartisan Commission has made a similar calculation (National Bipartisan Commission 1999a). The commission's calculation also shows the FEHBP outperforming private-sector employers but not the most similar competitive program, operated by the state of California for its employees.

The earliest calculation, for 1986–1995, reflects years when Medicare had just implemented the prospective payment system for hospitals. Medicare was paying hospitals well below actual cost and was shifting hospital costs onto private sector plans, including those in the FEHBP (see Francis 1993a). Both plans and OPM overestimated cost increases in the early 1990s and raised premiums too high (excess revenues went into trust fund reserves).

The latest ten-year calculation, covering 1990–1999, reflects years during which the FEHBP radically shifted toward managed care, with HMO enrollment reaching 40 percent for employees and preferred-provider enrollment rising from nearly zero to almost all remaining employees (but not annuitants on Medicare).

During all years, three major trends have affected costs; one favored the FEHBP and competition, and two, Medicare and cost controls. First, the number of expensive federal annuitants older than sixty-five without Medicare coverage has been falling, as the oldest cohort of retirees dies (Medicare did not cover federal employees until 1983). Second, FEHBP plans have significantly improved benefits, while Medicare has not. Third, the federal work force has aged substantially, while Medicare enrollees are younger. Despite the adverse effect of the latter trends, the FEHBP has overcome Medicare's monopsonistic advantage and greatly reduced the rate of cost increase.

Clearly, some of this better performance reflects one-time savings accruing from the conversion to managed care. If managed care has reached the limit of possible savings, then the difference between the two programs would be expected to narrow. If, however, managed-care plans continue to realize additional savings through improved service delivery (for example, large-case management), efficiency (for example, switching to generic drugs), and payment policies, the FEHBP design may have a semi-permanent and increasing cost advantage over relatively unfettered fee-for-service medicine as practiced in Medicare.

**Benefit Performance.** A comparison of benefits is hardly fair. Traditional Medicare largely remains a relic of insurance design vintage 1960, with an artificial distinction between in- and outpatient care, an antiquated benefit structure, a huge hospital deductible, and tremendous coverage gaps. In contrast, the FEHBP has modernized deductibles, improved prescription-drug coverage, and improved catastrophic limits—virtually without controversy. Benefit supplementation (Medigap) plans are a virtual necessity in Medicare but are nonexistent in the FEHBP.

**Implementation and Administration.** There are few aspects of these programs in which OPM has not performed well or excelled, and many aspects in which the Health Care Financing Administration (HCFA) has stumbled (Francis 1993a). After a dozen or more years of active HMO participation in Medicare, the program did not have such simple necessities as factual, organized, plain-English, or even available materials to enable beneficiaries to compare their choices of plans (GAO 1999, 1996). Any available materials are confusingly worded and sometimes erroneous (Fox et al. 1999).

The 1999 plan comparison guide (HCFA 1998) contains only ten information entries for each plan, including name, telephone number, premium, and copayments, compared with twenty-four entries for most plans in the equivalent OPM guide and almost twice as many for the national plans (OPM 1998). Current HCFA drafts for written information for the year 2000 would drop even this limited benefit and copayment information (albeit adding two quality measures) and would require seniors to contact plans individually to obtain basic benefit information. Meanwhile, as of spring 1999, the HCFA web site requires approximately sixty mouse clicks to view all information on the half-dozen HMOs in the typical state and dozens more to print the information. OPM mails requested brochures to each senior and allows on-line users to download a complete brochure, containing far more information, with one mouse click per plan. While HCFA intends to remedy some of these and other weaknesses, most seniors will, for at least several more years, find it difficult and time-consuming to obtain clear, comprehensive, and authoritative information on plan choices (Francis 1999).

**Premium Cost-Sharing.** Under the FEHBP, consumer incentives to select the best-buy plans, and plan incentives to restrain costs, are substantially attenuated because OPM cannot pay more than 75 percent of the cost of any plan. Even if a plan can deliver care at less than the maximum government contribution, there is little incentive to do so because the government captures 75 percent of any saving. (Feldman, Dowd, and Coulam, forthcoming, analyze this issue in more detail.) Medicare offers much higher incentives to many beneficiaries. For the one-third who pay their own Medigap premium, at an average cost of $1,300 a year (Congress 1998), enrolling in a low- or no-premium HMO with better hospital and medical benefits and prescription-drug coverage represents a major saving.

**Risk Selection and Risk Management.** There are several kinds of risk selection. First, there is the arguably desirable kind in which consumers sort themselves out by their differing preferences. The willingness to pay for these differences is disciplined by their cost; this would seem to be a natural and desirable variation for any product, including health insurance. When health insurance consumers select their own insurance plans, a felicitous result occurs: they naturally pool themselves. Each group pays the excess marginal cost of its preferences. So long as plans are priced fairly for the benefits that they provide, and protect against catastrophic expense and meet other standards, why should government care what specific benefits they offer? Equally important, plans that can vary benefits can evolve over time.

A second form of risk selection arises when differences in plan features, enrollment, and premiums reflect people sorting themselves out into more-sick and less-sick groups. HMOs have traditionally sought and attracted younger persons, because they cover pregnancy and well-baby visits at 100 percent, while older and sicker persons tend to stay in fee-for-service plans for better provider selection and access to specialists. Many consider such selection to be ethically offensive. However, we tolerate risk segmentation in most forms of insurance. For example, young persons pay much lower premiums for life insurance but much higher auto insurance premiums than older persons do. Age rating for premiums is ubiquitous in the individual and small-group health insurance market.

A third form of risk selection involves issues of moral hazard, where information asymmetries can lead to market failure. In the classic example, as sicker patients join a plan with better benefits, its premiums must rise to cover costs. Healthier patients join the plan with lower premiums. Over time, a "death spiral" occurs.

What about FEHBP and Medicare performance? The traditional Medicare program insists on identical benefits for all and identical premiums for all (leaving aside subsidies for the poor through the Medicaid program). There is no product variation, risk segmentation, or moral hazard. (The addition of HMO options has, of course, raised these issues.)

The FEHBP has much variation in minor benefits, which leads to many choices for consumers to exercise their preferences. There is also risk segmentation. Part of the continuing differential between HMO and fee-for-service premiums, for example, reflects the willingness of older and statistically sicker persons to pay more for greater provider choice. However, destructive death spirals have been almost absent from the program. Large and continuing premium disparities, even among fee-for-service plans with similar benefits, have continued for many years without death spirals. This stable record is all the more remarkable because there are several large and distinct risk groups within the program, such as a once-large cohort of elderly retirees without Medicare coverage. Perhaps this stability reflects the paradox that HMOs are "best buys" not only for the healthiest but also for the sickest.

The FEHBP has not been given tools for dealing with risk selection. The badly flawed formula of adjusted average per capita cost (AAPCC) did at least allow Medicare to vary its contribution to HMO premiums by age of enrollee. In the FEHBP, the existence of statistically predictable high-cost elderly persons without Medicare coverage cried out for a differential payment to plans, but the FEHBP had no power to adjust.

The FEHBP's only power to control risk selection lies in bargaining over potential benefit changes that might disadvantage specific higher-risk groups. To the credit of the plans and OPM, virtually no invidious benefit distinctions of this kind have been present in the program. This potential problem, which is central to arguments for standardizing benefits (Enthoven 1989; Fox et al. 1999), has simply not been observed in the program.

The FEHBP's lack of control mechanisms results in one major adverse consequence. The effects of risk segmentation on premiums distort and compromise the ability of enrollees to choose among plans because of benefit characteristics. For example, the Blue Cross high option has long had the most generous outpatient mental health benefit in the program. Because most enrollees in that plan are elderly persons without Medicare, a younger enrollee must choose both the mental health coverage and the expensive enrollment group.

**Locus of Decision.** There is a more fundamental distinction between the programs that cost, benefit, and risk-selection comparisons merely reflect. In the FEHBP, the locus of decisionmaking ultimately rests with individual consumers. The plans, and hence the program, adjust dynamically to these decisions in an almost transparent fashion. In Medicare, the locus of decisionmaking is the political process (Can 1999). The federal political process has been driven over the past decade by the need to find budgetary savings. Otherwise, it seeks to avoid inflicting transitory pain. By preserving what exists, it precludes improvement. The failure to reform HMO reimbursement (the AAPCC was finally addressed but only partially reformed in the Balanced Budget Act of 1997) delayed by a decade the ability of millions of elderly beneficiaries to obtain low-cost prescription-drug coverage and gap-free catastrophic coverage. The FEHBP's failures are most acute where it is most constrained by law, for example, in the absence of tools for risk management, in denying new fee-for-service plan entry, and (until a recent reform) in erroneously calculating the all-plan average premium.

Further, because the FEHBP allows benefit variations, the political process finds no simple target for change (or, more likely, refusal to change) through political rather than market processes. Precisely because the FEHBP does not have one-size-fits-all deductibles, coinsurance rates, payment mechanisms, provider participation, and coverage limitations, parochial interests and budget cutters have relatively few fixed points to either attack or defend. Medicare, in constrast, is a micromanager's delight (there are about fifty changes to Medicare law each year, according to Cain 1999).

## Moving Medicare toward the FEHBP Model

Medicare is already on the road toward a competitive system. Particularly with the reforms enacted in the Balanced Budget Act of 1997, HMOs will sooner or later have a realistic opportunity to compete for enrollment throughout the country. These reforms include stability of payment rates and enrollment decisions (enrollees will no longer be able to shift between plans more than once a year), availability of comparative information, and other essential ingredients of working markets. The rapid growth in HMO participation and enrollment, up to about 300 plans and 14 percent of beneficiaries in 1997, is testimony to the desire of beneficiaries for such choices (Congress 1998). Even the 1998 pullout of some fifty HMOs over a rate dispute with HCFA and the 1999 pullouts over continuing problems with HMO reimbursement levels seem to reflect teething pains rather than real slowing in the evolution of the program. The failure of any fee-for-service or PPO plans to enlist in the program suggests that the statutory and regulatory barriers are too high for these plans. The main statutory impediment is a requirement that these plans meet the benefit structure of traditional Medicare. Also, until recent corrections of the most egregious clauses, codified rules for the Medicare+Choice program imposed almost insuperable barriers to PPO and fee-for-service plans.

In statutory, regulatory, institutional, and behavioral terms, the traditional Medicare program remains so preeminent that the likelihood of a natural evolution to a structure that closely resembles the FEHBP is low. What, then, can be learned from the FEHBP about how a more fundamental reform could work? What pitfalls lurk, and how might they be avoided? How could the elderly be assured that neither benefits nor premiums would change substantially to their disadvantage?

**Premium Cost-Sharing.** Most Medicare beneficiaries pay only one-fourth of the Part B premium—$550 per person in 1999. This is about 10 percent of the total Part A and B cost. However, Medigap coverage of one kind or another (through enrollee, employer, or Medicaid) is paid for almost 90 percent of beneficiaries, at an average cost of $1,300 (Congress 1998) and rising rapidly. As a result, the direct taxpayer portion of total insurance costs is only about 75 percent, roughly the same as in the FEHBP.

Complicating the issue is the peculiar role of Medigap plans. (Benefit supplementation, except for dental care, is not needed in the FEHBP and virtually does not exist.) It is hard to imagine additional reforms in the Medicare program so imperfect that Medigap plans would still meet a real need or have a viable role.

These data suggest that creativity will be needed in premium design if Medicare attempts to implement a competitive system placing the marginal cost of decisions on enrollees without greatly changing underlying contribution shares. Should Medicare provide for rebates if some HMOs can deliver care for less than the average Medicare cost? How can premium shares be structured to avoid artificial windfalls or penalties for enrollees in plans with different cost structures (Merlis 1999)? Can employer subsidies for Medigap be grandfathered into the program rather than returned to employers as a windfall saving?

**Premium Growth.** Both the FEHBP and Medicare tie growth to actual changes in the cost of health care delivery for enrollees. For Medicare, this makes budget games and cost controls irresistible. The FEHBP's approach of tying premium growth to changes in the next year's insurance costs creates a smaller but substantial incentive for government to tinker with benefits to meet budgetary goals. Because Medicare is more than ten times the size of the FEHBP in dollar terms and has a tradition of budgetary tinkering, this does not augur well for reform. Ideally, the government share of premium growth should be decoupled from benefit decisions by enrollees and plans. Unfortunately, doing so would counter another important goal: ensuring that a reformed system does not tilt unduly toward higher costs on enrollees. This dilemma might be resolved by adjusting premiums based on a rolling average covering several years of costs. Annual changes in benefits would have an attenuated effect on the next year's budget.

Perhaps only a portion of the benefit package might count toward determination of the programwide average premium. The required minimum actuarial benefit discussed below might be set at 80 percent, with 90 percent as the maximum allowable for premium determination. Plans could add benefits without affecting the program's budget. A related solution, already used by the FEHBP, allows plans to add certain benefits (for example, hearing aids, dental care), with the entire cost borne offbudget by enrollees, not as part of the negotiated premium.

**Defining the Benefit Package.** Perhaps the most vocal concern of defenders of the present Medicare program has been the fear of losing particular benefit guarantees exhaustively described in law. Such a freeze, however, prevents consumer-driven evolution, innovations in cost control, and plan responsiveness to consumer preferences. This apparent dilemma should be one of the easiest to address. Benefits could be tied to actuarial measures of performance, similar to those used informally by OPM. Each plan could be required to have a benefit package that actuaries agree would pay not less than $X$ percent of hospital, medical, and prescription-drug costs faced by Medicare enrollees, where $X$ would be better than traditional Medicare. (Special rules could accommodate medical savings accounts or other unique cases.) The administering agency could be empowered to reject benefit gaps that would likely penalize enrollees or would foster undesirable risk selection.

Another argument for enumerating standardized benefits is the potential confusion of seniors. However, availability, accuracy, and clarity of benefit descriptions appear to be the major problems. Standardization would inhibit innovation (Fox et al. 1999).

**Risk Management.** Age-adjusted capitation rates as used in Medicare are an improvement over the nonexistent risk adjustments used in the FEHBP. Health-status risk adjustment will soon be added to Medicare as required by the Balanced Budget Act of 1997. But additional mechanisms could be used. Retrospective adjustments in government contributions to each plan could be made by pooling high-cost cases. Such a reinsurance mechanism would be particularly important for smaller plans but would also help with the problem that no risk adjusters predict costs with great precision.

The main lesson from the FEHBP is that the system as a whole will tolerate minimally adequate risk adjusters and much risk segmentation without destructive death spirals or real or perceived inequity. Medicare experience with AAPCC suggests that overcompensating for risk differences may be as much a problem as the opposite.

**The Future of Traditional Medicare.** The Breaux-Thomas proposal contemplates the continuation of traditional Medicare, competing with other plans for enrollment. Opponents fear that Medicare, overpriced through risk selection, would become the only option available in rural areas, to the detriment especially of the neediest elderly. Further, unless modified to include prescription drugs, Medicare might not be able to compete. Other problems include the inability to use panels of preferred providers and the uniform Part B premium. There is no simple answer to these concerns.

The difficulty millions of impoverished elderly have in paying premiums today is an issue, regardless of program model. Perhaps income tax credits could improve on the imperfect approach that relies on Medicaid agencies to find and subsidize the needy elderly. But that decision does not rest on the program model.

As argued below, the simplest remedy for malfunctioning in a newly redesigned program is careful monitoring, with further changes as needed. Suppose that the reform did not attract competing FFS-PPO plans. Entry into the program could be eased. Suppose that risk selection raised the cost of traditional Medicare in rural areas. A premium cross-subsidy could be imposed.

Traditional Medicare could be given limited authority to enrich some benefits while reducing others within circumscribed limits. A higher deductible could be combined with limited prescription-drug coverage. Concerns over price controls on prescription drugs could be met by requiring reliance on third-party contractors to design and administer the program. Premiums could vary modestly by geographic area. Traditional Medicare could be authorized to compete with other plans without an act of Congress for each benefit change.

**Implementation and Administration.** The Breaux-Thomas proposal would set up the new program under the auspices of a new Medicare board empowered to set standards, approve benefits, and negotiate premiums (National Bipartisan Commission 1999b). This structure reflects the view that HCFA would be too conflicted if it were simultaneously in charge of the traditional program and acting as the referee for its competitors. In fact, some argue vigorously that no new program could succeed under HCFA administration (Cain 1999). A further jurisdictional problem arises because HCFA has evolved into a major regulatory agency with broad powers over most sectors of the health care system, quite apart from its responsibility for administering traditional Medicare.

HCFA, unlike OPM, has a record of failing to handle its responsibilities for competitive plan oversight with careful attention to problems and rapid development of solutions that facilitate constructive program evolution. An immense increase in responsibilities and in the complexity of the program has been imposed on HCFA in recent years without attendant increases in resources. But their institutional problem is clearly more fundamental, as is the failure of HCFA to adopt simple and inexpensive pro-consumer and pro-choice information practices similar to those long used by OPM.

**Evolution.** If the test for adoption of the FEHBP as a model for Medicare is absolute certainty that today's design decisions will avoid all major problems over decades, the test must inevitably be failed. If the problem is approached from the perspective that the reformed program can be modified when and if and to the extent that particular problems emerge, then the FEHBP model—suitably improved to correct known defects—offers a reasonable path to at least modest, and possibly substantial, gains in the equity, efficiency, and adequacy of benefits.

## References

American Medical Association. 1995. *Transforming Medicare*. Washington, D.C.: AMA.

Anderson, Odin, and J. Joel May. 1971. "The Federal Employees Health Benefits Program, 1961–68: A Model for National Health Insurance?" In *Perspectives*. Chicago: Center for Health Administration Studies, University of Chicago.

Board of Trustees of the Federal Hospital Insurance Trust Fund. 1999. *Annual Report of the Federal Hospital Insurance Trust Fund*. Washington, D.C.: Government Printing Office.

Butler, Stuart, and Robert Moffit. 1995. "The FEHBP as a Model for a New Medicare Program." *Health Affairs* 14 (4).

Cain, Harry P. II. 1999. "Moving Medicare to the FEHBP Model, or How to Make an Elephant Fly." *Health Affairs* 18 (4).

Enthoven, Alain C. 1989. "Management of Competition in the FEHBP." *Health Affairs 8* (3) (fall).

———. 1980. *Health Plan: The Only Practical Solution to the Soaring Cost of Medical Care*. Reading, Mass.: Addison-Wesley.

Feldman, Roger, Bryan Dowd, and Robert Coulam. forthcoming. "The Federal Employees Health Benefits Plan: Implications for Medicare Reform." Minneapolis: Division of Health Services Research and Policy, University of Minnesota.

Fox, Peter D., Rani Snyder, Geraldine Dalleck, and Thomas Rice. 1999. "Should Medicare Benefits Be Standardized?" *Health Affairs* 18 (4).

Francis, Walton. 1999. Testimony on Medicare+Choice, Subcommittee on Health, Committee on Ways and Means, House of Representatives, U.S. Congress, March 18.

———. 1993a. "The Political Economy of the Federal Employees Health

Benefits Program." In *Health Policy Reform: Competition and Controls*, edited by Robert B. Helms. Washington, D.C.: AEI Press.

———. 1993b. "A Health Care Program Run by the Government That Works." *The American Enterprise*, July–August.

Merck, Carolyn. 1999. "The Medicare Program and the Federal Employees Health Benefits Program: Purpose, Design, and Operations." Congressional Research Service Report for Congress. Washington, D.C.

Merlis, Mark. 1999. *Medicare Restructuring: The FEHBP Model*. Menlo Park, Calif.: Henry J. Kaiser Family Foundation.

National Bipartisan Commission on the Future of Medicare. 1999a. "Fiscal Analysis of Senator Breaux's Premium Support Proposal." Meeting agenda of February 24. At http://rs9.loc.gov/medicare.

———. 1999b. "Draft Working Document." January 21. At http://rs9.loc.gov/medicare.

Schmid, Stuart. 1995. "Geographic Variation in Medical Costs: Evidence from HMOs." *Health Affairs* 14 (1) (spring).

Thorpe, Kenneth, Curtis S. Florence, Bradley Gray, and Katherine Harris. Forthcoming. *Does Design Matter? The Impact of the Federal Employees Health Benefits (FEHB) Program on Plan Premiums, Plan Choice and Subscriber Satisfaction*. New Orleans: Tulane University Medical Center.

U.S. Congress, House of Representatives, Committee on Ways and Means. 1998. *1998 Green Book*. Washington, D.C.: Government Printing Office.

U.S. General Accounting Office. 1996. *HCFA Should Release Data to Aid Consumers, Prompt Better HMO Performance*. Washington, D.C.: Government Printing Office.

———. 1999. *Medicare+Choice: New Standards Could Improve Accuracy and Usefulness of Plan Literature*. Washington, D.C.: Government Printing Office.

U.S. Health Care Financing Administration. 1998. *Medicare and You 1999*. Washington, D.C.: Government Printing Office.

U.S. Office of Personnel Management. 1998. *1999 Guide to Federal Employees Health Benefits Plans*. Washington, D.C.: Government Printing Office.

Vladek, Bruce. 1999. "The Political Economy of Medicare." *Health Affairs* 18 (1) (January–February).

# Index

## Board of Trustees

Edward B. Rust, Jr., *Chairman*
Chairman and CEO
State Farm Insurance Companies

Tully M. Friedman, *Treasurer*
Chairman
Friedman Fleischer & Lowe, LLC

Joseph A. Cannon
Chairman and CEO
Geneva Steel Company

Dick Cheney
CEO
Halliburton Company

Harlan Crow
Chief Executive Officer
Crow Holdings

Christopher C. DeMuth
President
American Enterprise Institute

Steve Forbes
President and CEO
Forbes Inc.

Christopher B. Galvin
CEO
Motorola, Inc.

Harvey Golub
Chairman and CEO
American Express Company

Robert F. Greenhill
Chairman
Greenhill & Co., LLC

Roger Hertog
President and COO
Sanford C. Bernstein and Company

M. Douglas Ivester
Chairman and CEO
The Coca-Cola Company

Martin M. Koffel
Chairman and CEO
URS Corporation

Bruce Kovner
Chairman
Caxton Corporation

Kenneth L. Lay
Chairman and CEO
Enron Corp.

John A. Luke, Jr.
Chairman, President, and CEO
Westvaco Corporation

Alex J. Mandl
Chairman and CEO
Teligent, Inc.

Craig O. McCaw
Chairman and CEO
Eagle River, Inc.

Paul H. O'Neill
Chairman and CEO
Alcoa

John E. Pepper
Chairman
The Procter & Gamble Company

George R. Roberts
Kohlberg Kravis Roberts & Co.

John W. Rowe
Chairman, President, and CEO
Unicom Corporation

James P. Schadt
Chairman
Dailey Capital Management

John W. Snow
Chairman, President, and CEO
CSX Corporation

William S. Stavropoulos
Chairman and CEO
The Dow Chemical Company

Wilson H. Taylor
Chairman and CEO
CIGNA Corporation

Marilyn Ware
Chairman
American Water Works Co., Inc.

James Q. Wilson
James A. Collins Professor of
Management Emeritus
University of California at Los
Angeles

## The American Enterprise Institute for Public Policy Research

Founded in 1943, AEI is a nonpartisan, nonprofit research and educational organization based in Washington, D. C. The Institute sponsors research, conducts seminars and conferences, and publishes books and periodicals.

AEI's research is carried out under three major programs: Economic Policy Studies; Foreign Policy and Defense Studies; and Social and Political Studies. The resident scholars and fellows listed in these pages are part of a network that also includes ninety adjunct scholars at leading universities throughout the United States and in several foreign countries.

The views expressed in AEI publications are those of the authors and do not necessarily reflect the views of the staff, advisory panels, officers, or trustees.

## Officers

Christopher C. DeMuth
President

David Gerson
Executive Vice President

John R. Bolton
Senior Vice President

## Council of Academic Advisers

James Q. Wilson, *Chairman*
James A. Collins Professor of
Management Emeritus
University of California at Los
Angeles

Gertrude Himmelfarb
Distinguished Professor of History
Emeritus
City University of New York

Samuel P. Huntington
Albert J. Weatherhead III University
Professor of Government
Harvard University

D. Gale Johnson
Eliakim Hastings Moore
Distinguished Service Professor of
Economics Emeritus
University of Chicago

William M. Landes
Clifton R. Musser Professor of
Economics
University of Chicago Law School

Sam Peltzman
Sears Roebuck Professor of
Economics and Financial Services
University of Chicago Graduate
School of Business

Nelson W. Polsby
Professor of Political Science
University of California at Berkeley

George L. Priest
John M. Olin Professor of Law and
Economics
Yale Law School

Thomas Sowell
Senior Fellow
Hoover Institution
Stanford University

Murray L. Weidenbaum
Mallinckrodt Distinguished
University Professor
Washington University

Paul Wolfowitz
Dean, Paul H. Nitze School of
Advanced International Studies
Johns Hopkins University

Richard J. Zeckhauser
Frank Ramsey Professor of Political
Economy
Kennedy School of Government
Harvard University

## Research Staff

Leon Aron
Resident Scholar

Claude E. Barfield
Resident Scholar; Director, Science
and Technology Policy Studies

Walter Berns
Resident Scholar

Douglas J. Besharov
Resident Scholar

Robert H. Bork
John M. Olin Scholar in Legal
Studies

Karlyn Bowman
Resident Fellow

Ricardo Caballero
Visiting Scholar

John E. Calfee
Resident Scholar

Charles Calomiris
Visiting Scholar

Lynne V. Cheney
Senior Fellow

Dinesh D'Souza
John M. Olin Research Fellow

Nicholas N. Eberstadt
Visiting Scholar

Mark Falcoff
Resident Scholar

Gerald R. Ford
Distinguished Fellow

Murray F. Foss
Visiting Scholar

Hillel Fradkin
Resident Fellow

Diana Furchtgott-Roth
Assistant to the President and
Resident Fellow

Suzanne Garment
Visiting Scholar

Jeffrey Gedmin
Resident Scholar; Executive Director,
New Atlantic Initiative

Newt Gingrich
Senior Fellow

James K. Glassman
DeWitt Wallace–Reader's Digest
Fellow

Robert A. Goldwin
Resident Scholar

Robert W. Hahn
Resident Scholar; Director,
AEI–Brookings Joint Center for
Regulatory Studies

Kevin Hassett
Resident Scholar

Tom Hazlett
Resident Scholar

Robert B. Helms
Resident Scholar; Director, Health
Policy Studies

R. Glenn Hubbard
Visiting Scholar

James D. Johnston
Resident Fellow

Leon Kass
W. H. Brady, Jr., Scholar

Jeane J. Kirkpatrick
Senior Fellow; Director, Foreign and
Defense Policy Studies

Marvin H. Kosters
Resident Scholar; Director, Economic
Policy Studies

Irving Kristol
John M. Olin Distinguished Fellow

Michael A. Ledeen
Freedom Scholar

James Lilley
Resident Fellow

Lawrence Lindsey
Arthur F. Burns Scholar in
Economics

Clarisa Long
Abramson Fellow

Randall Lutter
Resident Scholar

John H. Makin
Visiting Scholar; Director, Fiscal
Policy Studies

Allan H. Meltzer
Visiting Scholar

James M. Morris
Director of Publications

Joshua Muravchik
Resident Scholar

Charles Murray
Bradley Fellow

Michael Novak
George F. Jewett Scholar in Religion,
Philosophy, and Public Policy;
Director, Social and Political Studies

Norman J. Ornstein
Resident Scholar

Richard N. Perle
Resident Fellow

Sarath Rajapatirana
Visiting Scholar

William Schneider
Resident Scholar

J. Gregory Sidak
F. K. Weyerhaeuser Fellow

Christina Hoff Sommers
W. H. Brady, Jr., Fellow

Herbert Stein
Senior Fellow

Daniel Troy
Associate Scholar

Arthur Waldron
Visiting Scholar; Director, Asian
Studies

Graham Walker
Visiting Scholar

Peter Wallison
Resident Fellow

Ben J. Wattenberg
Senior Fellow

Carolyn L. Weaver
Resident Scholar; Director, Social
Security and Pension Studies

David Wurmser
Research Fellow

Karl Zinsmeister
J. B. Fuqua Fellow; Editor,
*The American Enterprise*

*This book was edited by
Ann Petty of the American Enterprise Institute.
The index was prepared by Julia Petrakis.
The text was set in Bodoni.
Cynthia Stock, Electronic Quill,
of Silver Spring, Maryland, set the type,
and Edwards Brothers, Incorporated,
of Lillington, North Carolina,
printed and bound the book,
using permanent acid-free paper.*

The AEI Press is the publisher for the American Enterprise Institute for Public Policy Research, 1150 Seventeenth Street, N.W., Washington, D.C. 20036. *Christopher DeMuth,* publisher; *James Morris,* director; *Ann Petty,* editor; *Leigh Tripoli,* editor; *Cheryl Weissman,* editor; *Kenneth Krattenmaker,* art director and production manager; *Jean-Marie Navetta,* production assistant.